Greek Medical Manuscripts
Diels' Catalogue

Tome 3: Corpus Galenicum

Medical Traditions

Edited by
Alain Touwaide

Volume 2/3

De Gruyter

Greek Medical Manuscripts
Diels' Catalogue

Tome 3: Corpus Galenicum

Newly revised and updated by
Alain Touwaide

De Gruyter

ISBN 978-3-11-060068-1
e-ISBN (PDF) 978-3-11-060004-9
ISSN 2567-6938

Library of Congress Control Number: 2020945916

Bibliographic information published by the Deutsche Nationalbibliothek
The Deutsche Nationalbibliothek lists this publication in the Deutsche Nationalbibliografie; detailed bibliographic data are available on the Internet at http://dnb.dnb.de.

Cover image: Collage of illustrations in medical treatises from the 1st to the 16th century CE, from Greece and Rome, to the Arabic World and China.

Printing: CPI books GmbH, Leck

www.degruyter.com

Table of contents

Foreword

The study of Greek manuscripts of medical content has seen a significant, though not exclusive, investigation by Alain Touwaide, whose life of scholar has been entirely devoted to the knowledge and valorization of the medical traditions of the Mediterranean world with a particular reference to the history of ancient and medieval Greek medicine.

The revisions and updates of the catalogues of Greek medical manuscripts compiled in the early 20th century by an équipe of philologists, guided by the distinguished historian of ancient Greek philosophy and medicine Hermann Diels (*Die Handschriften der antiken Ärzte*), are a cornerstone of Touwaide's scientific research on medical manuscripts, the further developments of which already include plans for a detailed catalogue of all surviving witnesses according to the norms of modern catalography.

Four years after his 2016 voluminous *Census of Greek Medical Manuscripts*, the publication of this new and substantial reference work constitutes a further step, complementary to the previous one, of his programme that will ultimately allow for the critical edition of a series of Greek medical texts in a way reminiscent of the *Corpus Medicorum* conceived by Diels over a century ago as the natural outcome of the catalogues of manuscripts that he coordinated.

If Alain Touwaide embarked on an arduous task with his *Census* and the compilation of an updated list of Greek manuscripts with medical contents—many of which were not listed in Diels' early 20th-century catalogues—the completion of a renewed Diels is a no less demanding endeavour. Diels' catalogues, which have been the reference for over a century for any scholar interested in the study of late antique and medieval Greek medicine from any perspective, are known, indeed, to suffer several limitations—besides the incompleteness of their inventory of manuscripts (well highlighted by the numerous complements provided in the *Census*)—that can be traced to the difficulty in identifying manuscripts generated by Diels' use of shelfmarks which have been made obsolete since by changes in the name of libraries or collections, in ownership, or in the location of collections. To further make research laborious, the printing of Diels' original edition is rather unclear.

Alain Touwaide has chosen to exactly reproduce the substance of Diels' work, even though he significantly intervened with great acumen on the structure, citation format, and presentation of the text, to make its contents more immediately usable and its consultation easier. An innovative organization of data in five tomes (in which the reproduction of Diels' original text in a decidedly more readable form is followed by two different methods of accessing the information, by type of contents—in tomes two through four—and by manuscript—in the fifth and final tome) is accompanied by an articulated system of indices designed to combine the need to reproduce Diels' original text *ad litteram* and the scientific imperative to update and standardize the method of referencing the manuscripts, and also to multiply the keys for searching the texts. In this view, Touwaide's decision to split the list of authors and works is revealing as it allows for the identification of texts by both their Greek and Latin title (albeit following the form, which is not always consistent, of the titles in Diels' original version), thus providing a first effort for a future standardization. Equally inspired by a justifiable need for clarity and simplification is the choice of accompanying the index of the original shelfmarks of manuscripts with a list of the English names of the cities and libraries. Finally, the layout of this renewed Diels clearly improves on the original edition, structuring its presentation in a much clearer and more effective way through different levels of indentation.

Those who are acquainted with Alain Touwaide know that only his visionary and tenacious spirit, supported by an unshakable patience and a truly extraordinary work capacity, could have pushed him to embark alone on the revision of the catalogues that Diels conceived and could complete thanks to the collaboration of a team of no fewer than thirty scholars. Touwaide's revision required many long years of meticulous work, with a sheer quantity of doublechecks, corrections, and identifications of new locations and shelfmarks, as well as *in situ* autoptic inspection of many manuscripts and sometimes even of entire collections.

Though constantly making explicit its connection with Diels' original work through its coherent and functional system of cross-references, the present revision of Diels will ultimately make it unnecessary to refer to the old Diels and make it possible, instead, to work only with updated lists of manuscripts. Furthermore, the multiple indices extremely well designed by Touwaide and the cross-referencing they make possible pave the way to a future, highly desirable transfer of data from a printed form to an open database, much of the necessary material of which is contained in the present work, in addition to the new data already provided by the *Census*. It can be expected that such a database will be constantly expanded and updated by integrating the results of the new developments and research that the catalogue that we have here will undoubtedly contribute to, promote, and generate.

The renewed Diels that we have here deserves to be hailed as an invaluable reference for both the niche of scholars scrutinizing Greek medical manuscripts and texts, and the wider circle of the historians of medicine, pharmacy, and ancient and medieval science, in a way that faithfully reflects the cross-disciplinary approach to the study of medical traditions that Alain Touwaide has convincingly advocated for for years in the name of a fruitful alliance of sciences and the humanities.

We now wish that, as a further contribution to the knowledge of the ancient Greek medical tradition, he will publish a much needed catalogue of Greek medical manuscripts and texts, not only those listed in Diels, but also the many new ones of which he has revealed the existence thanks to his unwavering energy, his devotion to research, and the passion for Greek medicine that has constantly distinguished his life.

Marilena Maniaci
Università degli Studi di Cassino e del Lazio meridionale
Rome, August 2, 2020

Introduction

Just over a century has passed since a team of scholars from across Europe, led by German historian of ancient philosophy and science Hermann Diels (1848–1922)[1], compiled the manuscripts containing Greek medical texts and their medieval translations into a catalogue[2]. Following such classical bibliographies as the *Bibliotheca Graeca* by Johann Albert Fabricius (1668–1736)[3] and the several *Bibliothecae* by Albrecht von Haller (1708–1777)[4], *Diels*, as the catalogue became known, was a landmark in classical and medico-historical scholarship[5]. It was not completely

1 For a broad approach to Diels' multifaceted activity, see for example Calder et al. 1999. All works referred to in this introduction are cited in an abbreviated form (author's last name and year of publication). For the full reference, see the bibliography at pp. xxi–xxx.

2 The catalogue was published in two issues in 1905 and 1906, in the proceedings of Berlin Academy of Science, with a supplement in 1908 in the same series (Diels 1905, 1906a, and 1908, respectively). The 1905 and 1906 issues were published together as a volume in 1906 (Diels 1906b) with a slightly different title (*Die Handschriften der antiken Ärzte, Griechische Abteilung*) which implied that a similar programme would have dealt with the Latin manuscripts. The frontmatter of the second issue (1906a), which provided a general presentation of the programme, the list of the collaborators, and the bibliography, is reproduced as the front matter of this volume with the same pagination as in the first publication. All three issues (1905, 1906a, and 1908) were reprinted in 1970 with an introduction by Fridolf Kudlien (1928–2008) (Kudlien 1970). The translations under consideration were those in Syriac, Arabic, Hebrew, and Latin according to the treatises.
All references to the catalogue here and in the present work comprise two elements: the first identifies the issue of the catalogue (I, II, or N [for *Nachtrag* = Supplement]), and the second (in Arabic numerals) provides the number of the page(s) referred to (e.g., I.22 or N.49). A number in Arabic numerals between parentheses after the second element, such as e.g., II.63 (2), indicates the number of mentions of a manuscript on the same page.

3 Fabricius' *Bibliotheca Graeca* was originally published in 14 volumes between 1705 and 1728, with a second edition started as early as 1708 and pursued until 1754, and also a third edition of Volumes 1 and 2 published in 1718 and 1752, respectively. The whole *Bibliotheca* was further published in a revised edition by Gottlieb Christopher Harles (1738–1815) in 12 volumes published between 1790 and 1809, with an *Index* in 1838. Under the general designation *Bibliotheca Graeca*, all volumes have a distinctive title that indicates their respective contents. In the first volume this title makes an explicit reference to manuscripts (... *notitia Scriptorum Veterum Graecorum quorumcunque monumenta integra, aut fragmenta edita exstant: tum plerorumque è MSS. ac deperditis* ...). On Fabricius, see Verner 1966.

4 The first of Haller's *Bibliothecae* was the *Bibliotheca botanica* (1771–1772), which included large chapters on ancient physicians (see for example, Dioscorides, vol. 1, pp. 79–87 [page 79 is numbered 97]). It was followed by the *Bibliotheca chirurgica* (1774–1775), the *Bibliotheca anatomica* (1774–1777), and the *Bibliotheca medicinae practicae* (1776–1788).

5 For the history of the search for the manuscripts of Greek medical texts from the Renaissance to Diels, see Touwaide 2009, particularly pp. 456–508.

unprecedented, however. From the late eighteenth century on, several similar compilations were made, indeed, but they relied either on earlier literature or on *in situ* inspection of just some collections by single scholars. These were the bibliographies compiled by Johann Christian Gottlieb Ackermann (1756–1801)[6] and the pioneering search for manuscripts by the German scholar Friedrich Reinhold Dietz (1804–1836) in the 1830s[7], followed shortly after by the exploratory missions of the French historian of medicine Charles Daremberg (1817–1872), mostly in England[8], with a similar collection of material *in loco* at the Bibliothèque nationale in Paris by the Greek ophthalmologist Georges Costomiris (1849–1902)[9]. Diels' enterprise was different in its systematicity and scale, in addition to its organization, its team[10], and its international network[11] which combined in-house bibliographical research[12] and *in-*

6 Ackermann's bibliographies with their lists of manuscripts for Hippocrates, Dioscorides and Galen, were published in Harles' edition of Fabricius' *Bibliotheca Graeca* (vol. 2 [1791], pp. 506–611, 4 [1795], pp. 673–702, and 5 [1796], pp. 377–500, respectively). The lists of Hippocratic and Galenic manuscripts were reproduced in the edition of these authors in Kühn's *Medicorum Graecorum Opera quae exstant* under the title *Historia literaria* (for Hippocrates, see vol. 1 [1825], pp. I–CCVI; for Galen, see vol. 1 [1821]), pp. XIX–CCLXV). Interestingly enough, Diels referred to these two lists. The list of manuscripts for Dioscorides, *De materia medica*, in Kühn's *Medicorum Graecorum Opera quae exstant* (see vol. 1 [1829], pp. XX–XXVI) did not reproduce Ackermann's, but was compiled by the editor of the text, Kurt Sprengel (1766–1833).

7 Dietz traveled through Germany, Italy, Spain, France, and Britain, systematically searching for codices containing Greek medical texts (see Dietz 1832: IX–X; Dietz 1834: 1.IV), principally Hippocrates, but also Oribasius (he was supposed to prepare an edition for the corpus edited by Kühn), Aetius, the commentators on Hippocrates, Ioannes Zacharias Actuarius, Greek chemical works, Soranus, Paul of Aegina, Rufus of Ephesus, Erotianus, Nicander, Theophilus, Symeon Seth, and others (e.g., Severus iatrosophist whose treatise he published [Dietz 1836]).

8 See the reports of his travels in Daremberg 1845, 1848, 1851, and 1852, with a reproduction of the last two in the form of a monograph in 1853.

9 Costomiris published the results of his investigations at the Bibliothèque nationale in a series of five contributions to the *Revue des études grecques* published between 1889 and 1897.

10 The collaborators of the program are listed in the front matter of the 1906 issue and the 1906 reprint (p. X) with some further names in the 1908 supplement (p. 23). Besides the collaborators *in loco* (among whom were Ph.D. candidates) coordinated in collaboration by Diels and Johan Ludwig Heiberg (1854–1928), the team included several German scholars as Joseph Heeg (1881–1916) in Munich, Georg Helmreich (1849–1921) in Ansbach, Johannes Ilberg (1860–1930) in Leipzig, Karl Kalbfleich (1868–1946) in Marburg, Iwan von Müller (1830–1917) at that time in Munich, Paul Schwarz (1867–1938), then in Berlin, and Max Wellmann (1863–1933). Their number was higher, however, as the reading of the catalogues indicates: the annotations that accompany the mention of some manuscripts refer to scholars whose name does not appear in the two lists of collaborators.

11 The list of collaborators includes several individuals from abroad who were librarians or academics with a special interest in the history of ancient medicine and medical literature, including translations. These scholars were the following (in alphabetical order of last name): Hartwig (Henry) Derembourg (1844–1908) in Paris; Eduard Gottlob (1856–1922) in Krems a.

situ examination of entire library collections by local scholars or members of Diels' team in mission abroad[13].

Remarkably enough, the vast collection of data contained in the two issues of Diels' catalogues was assembled in barely four years[14], witnessing an exceptional mobilization of efforts and resources[15]. Although a supplement—presented as the first—was published in 1908, it was not followed by any other. Shortly after, the team lost some of its collaborators in the First World War[16], and the systematic search for the manuscripts of ancient medical texts was no longer pursued. Nevertheless, several

---

d. Donau; Montague Rhodes James (1862–1936) in Cambridge; Philip Christian Molhuysen (1870–1944) in Leiden; Alessandro Olivieri (1872–1950) in Naples; Adriano Piccolomini (1843–1907) in Cesena; Anton Ritter von Premerstein (1869–1935) in Vienna; Hans Raeder (1859–1969) in Copenhagen; Walter Scott (1855–1925) in Oxford, with a parenthesis in Montreal (1905–1908); Hermann Schöne (1870–1941) in Basel; Rezső Vári (1867–1940) in Budapest, and Eric Otto Windstedt (1880–1955) in Oxford. This list is not exhaustive, however, as other names appear scattered in the catalogues. The different collaborators interacted as the references to collations (see below) indicate.

12 The consulted bibliography (listed in the 1906a issue [pp. XI–XXIII] with a supplement in 1908 [pp. 23–24]) does not account for the full extent of the library resources consulted by the collaborators of the catalogues, which contain scattered references to works not included in the bibliographical lists.

13 One such mission was that of Max Wellmann, who spent 1906–1907 in Italy, where he particularly investigated the collections of the Vatican and the Marciana libraries. As a result, the 1908 supplement contains multiple annotations made on the basis of his personal consultation of manuscripts.

14 To give an idea of the sheer quantity of data presented in the catalogues, suffice it to say that the number of items from Greek manuscripts only amounts to over 14,000. To this we should add the multiple collations of manuscripts made by the collaborators of the programme during *in loco* research stays or on their behalf that are mentioned in the catalogue. Ilberg, for example, collated himself or received collations of most of the Hippocratic writings from manuscripts at the Vatican Library, and in Florence, Venice, Vienna, and Paris, whereas Helmreich concentrated on Galen (in one case at least, he had a collation of all but one manuscript of a Galenic treatise; see I.83–84).

15 For the history of the programme, see Kollesch 1973, 1989, and 1999; and more recently, Nutton 2004.

16 This was the case of Bruno Rappaport (1875–1915), who managed the data of the catalogues in collaboration with Joahnnes Mewald (1880–1964). On this, see Diels' introductory remarks (*Vorbemerkungen*) to the catalogue (Diels 1906a: pp. I–IX), which include the reports by Rappaport (pp. III–VI) and Mewaldt (pp. VI–VIII). On Rappaport, see the obituary by Regling, 1920. Another victim of the First World War was Joseph Heeg. During the compilation of the catalogues, the program lost another of its members, the orientalist Ludwig Nix (1865–1904) who had collected much material about the Arabic translations of Greek medical works.

editions of Greek medical texts were published thanks to the material collected during the compiling of the catalogues[17].

Addenda and *corrigenda* to Diels[18], studies of the manuscripts or tradition of specific medical treatises[19], and the systematic inventory of the manuscripts of texts to be edited, with the analysis of their tradition[20], punctuated the twentieth-century scholarship devoted to the ancient medical literature. After World War II, an

17 The first such edition was that of Philumenus, *De venenatis animalibus*, by Max Wellmann who discovered the text in the manuscript *Vaticanus graecus* 284 during his research stay at the Vatican Library (Wellmann 1908). This edition, which inaugurated the *Corpus Medicorum Graecorum*, brilliantly illustrated the function of the catalogues as a source of firsthand material for the preparation of the critical editions to be published in the *Corpus*. It is probably significant that it was followed in 1914 by the edition of the Arabic translation of a Pseudo-Galenic treatise by Gotthelf Bergsträsser (1886–1933) (Bergsträsser 1914), and the first edition of Galen in the *Corpus* by three collaborators of the programme (Mewaldt et al. 1914). Another Galenic edition, prepared by another group of three collaborators, followed the next year (Diels et al. 1915), together with Celsus by Friedrich Marx (1869–1941) and, the following year, Quintus Serenus Sammonicus by Friedrich Vollmer (1867–1923). After a short interruption due to World War I, no fewer than 15 editions were published between 1921 and 1937, with one edition every year from 1926 on, including (in chronological order of publication) the vast medical encyclopedias of Paul of Aegina (Heiberg 1921–1924), Oribasius (Raeder 1926, and 1928–1933), and Aetius (*partim*; Olivieri, 1935), in addition to the first Hippocratic edition (Heiberg et al., 1927), Soranus (Ilberg, 1927), Galenic commentaries on Hippocratic treatises (Wenkebach 1934 and 1936) and Galenic works (Koch et al. 1923; De Boer 1937). All this attested to the vitality of the *Corpus* and the usefulness of the catalogue.

18 As early as 1916, Giovanni Mercati (1866–1957), then a *scrittore* at the Vatican Library, published some *addenda* (Mercati 1916, 1917a, and 1917b). Corrections like these are scattered throughout twentieth-century scholarly publications related to the Greek medical literature. Most of them can be found in Touwaide 2016, *passim*, together with new ones. Additions and corrections to Diels' lists of manuscripts of the Latin translations of Greek medical texts have been systematically made, though later. Richard Durling (1932–1999) revised Diels' lists of the Galenic Latin manuscripts (Durling 1967 and 1981, completed only recently by Fortuna and Raia 2006; a cumulative catalogue of the Galenic and Pseudo-Galenic Latin texts [including manuscripts] compiled by Stefania Fortuna and her group is now available online in the form of a constant work in progress [*Galeno. Catalogo delle traduzioni latine*]). Pearl Kibre (1902–1985) compiled new lists of the Hippocratic Latin manuscripts in several installments (1975–1982) followed by a publication in the form of a monographic catalogue in 1985. It may be relevant to note here that Durling expanded his search for Latin medical manuscripts by browsing a collection of material similar to Diels, Kristeller's *Iter Italicum* (Durling 1985–1993).

19 An early work of this type is Ilberg 1911 on Soranus, followed shortly after by Diels 1912 on Galen's commentary on Hippocrates *Prorrheticum*, and Helmreich 1913 on Symeon Seth.

20 The best examples are the introductions to the editions published in the *Corpus Medicorum Graecorum* (which became more developed over time). Their template includes a list of manuscripts, their description, and a detailed philological analysis. Although these introductions focus on identifying the manuscript(s) to be used as a source or sources of the editions, they provide relevant data on codicology and book history.

unprecedented increase in the interest in paleography and codicology[21] soon led to a renewed search for, and study of, manuscripts[22], new catalogues[23], and, more recently, computerized databases allowing for the storage and multi-criteria querying of increasingly larger amounts of information[24], in addition to the digitization of the collections of manuscripts of several libraries across the world[25]. In the field of Greek medical manuscripts and texts, this resulted in the rediscovery or, in some cases, in the true discovery of manuscripts[26], new catalogues of medical manuscripts[27], the history

21 In the field of Greek codicology and palaeography, and also textual history, this interest was pioneered by such scholars as Joseph Mogenet (1913–1980), Herbert Hunger (1914–2000), Jean Irigoin (1920–2006), and Paul Canart (1927–2017). It subsequently led to an increased institutionalization of these disciplines illustrated, among others, by a series of international conferences started in 1974 (see *Paléographie,* 1977). For a recent esquisse of the history of codicology and paleography during the twentieth century, see, for example, Touwaide 2010.

22 Whereas the type of research by Alphonse Dain (1896–1964), Paul Henry (1906–1984), Alexander Turyn (1900–1981), and Jean Irigoin on technical texts (Dain 1930, 1933, 1946), Plotin (Henry 1938, 1941), the Greek tragics (Turyn 1943, 1952, 1957) and Pindar (Turyn 1932, and Irigoin 1952), respectively, was relatively rare until then in the academic production, it became more common later. For examples of such a line of investigation, see Eleuteri 1981 on a literary text (Musaeus) and Sonderkamp 1987 on a Greek medical treatise (Theophanes Nonnos/Chrysobalantes).

23 The increase in the publication of catalogues of manuscripts can be best measured by comparing the successive editions of the so-called *Richard* (Richard 1948, 1958, and 1964, followed by such a punctual review of new catalogues as Irigoin 1970, and the major updated editions of *Richard* by Olivier 1995 and 2018).

24 One such database is PINAKES currently hosted and maintained by the Section Grecque of the Institut de Recherche et d'Histoire des Textes (IRHT) of the Centre National de la Recherche Scientifique (CNRS), in Paris. It is built on the basis of the earlier research conducted at the Pontifical Institute of Medieval Studies at University of Toronto by Robert E. Sinkewicz, who compiled available printed catalogues of manuscripts and published the resulting data in the form of microfiches (Sinkewicz and Hayes 1989; Sinkewicz 1990 and 1992). In the matter of medical manuscripts and texts, see the database built on Diels accessible online through the website of the Institute for the Preservation of Medical Traditions. A precursor of this type of database was the catalogue of incipits of Latin medical treatises compiled as early as 1937 by Lynn Thorndike (1882–1965) and Pearl Kibre (1937). After a revised edition published in 1963, this catalogue has been complemented by Linda E. Voigts and Patricia D. Kurtz (Voigts and Kurz 2004), and transformed in digital form (first as a CD-Rom and now as a database consultable online on the site of the University of Missouri Kansas City).

25 See, for example, the site *Gallica*, of the Bibliothèque nationale de France, *teca* of the Biblioteca Medicea Laurenziana in Firenze, *DVL-DigiVatLib* of the Vatican Library, *DigitalBodleian*, *Digitised Manuscripts* of the British Library or, to mention just some, *e-codices* for the manuscripts in Swiss collections. Significantly enough, the most recent release of the site of the *Corpus Medicorum Graecorum* includes links to the digital version of the manuscripts of the authors for which critical editions have been published in the *Corpus*.

26 The most spectacular case has been the discovery of the forgotten manuscript Thessaloniki, Vlatadon 14, which contains a Galenic text which had remained unknown thus far. See Pietrobelli, 2010, for example. For other cases, see, for example, Roselli 2009 ([Hippocrates]) or

of collections of such codices[28], an accrued attention to medical illustration[29], studies of the textual tradition of Greek medical texts[30] or genres[31], the medical production of some regions[32], and new critical editions, particularly from the mid-twentieth century onward[33]. This activity, which also generated a forum in the form of a series of conferences launched by Antonio Garzya (1927–2012) in 1990 and regularly held

---

Perilli 2011 (Galen's Hippocratic lexicon), and Chatzopoulou 2014 and Tselikas 2014 about *iatrosofia*.

27 For some catalogues, see Hunger and Kresten as early as 1969 about the series *medici graeci* of the National Library of Austria in Vienna, and, more recently, Bouras-Vallianatos 2015 about the holdings of the Wellcome Library in London, with a short supplement in Bouras-Vallianatos 2020. A different type of catalogue is that of Formentin 1978, about the libraries of a region.

28 See, for example, Formentin 1997 about the medical manuscripts in the collection of the national library in Naples.

29 A pioneering work in this field was MacKinney 1965, which lists the medieval manuscripts known at that time in several languages with medical illustrations, with some descriptive elements. Recently see Bernabò 2010.

30 For the entire tradition of some works, see, for example (in chronological order of publication), Kudlien 1960 (Hippocrates, *De articulis*), Rivier 1962 (Hippocrates, *De morbo sacro*), and Alexanderson 1963 (Hippocrates, *Prognosticon*) and 1967 (Galen, *De crisibus*). Among the studies in subsequent years, one might cite Morani 1981 (Nemesius) or, more recently, Perilli 1999 (Galen's Hippocratic lexicon). Similar work is being done in Latin, for example by Green 1996 and 1997, on *Trotula*. Research was also devoted to some lesser-known physicians such as Mercurius (see the study by Masullo 2006), or to some segments or manuscripts of the tradition of one or more works. This is the case of Wilson 1987, for example, regarding a group of Galenic manuscripts (the codices copied by Ioannikios), and Petit 2006 on a group of manuscripts in relation with a text ([Galen], *Introductio*).

31 For this type of catalogue, see, for example, Ihm 2002 on medical commentaries (with references to the manuscripts), or Karas 1994, and Tselikas 1995 on *iatrosophia* (Byzantine and later).

32 For Southern Italy, for example, see Ieraci Bio 1989.

33 After an interruption provoked by World War II, the *Corpus Medicorum Graecorum* published anew critical editions as early as 1950 with a predilection for Galen, also including, however, Hippocratic treatises, Aretaeus, Rufus of Ephesus, Aetius, and Leo medicus, and, more recently (from 1983 on), Stephanus of Athens and Johannes of Alexandria. In the 1960s, the French *Collection des universités de France* launched a new Hippocrates (see Joly 1978 for the first volume; the programme has been pursued by Jacques Jouanna) and, very recently, a new Galen (see Boudon 2000 for the first volume). All this in addition to editions in series specifically devoted to the history of ancient and medieval/Byzantine medicine as *Studies in Ancient Medicine* (for example, Dickson 1998 on Stephanus, and Zipser 2009 on Johannes archiater) or, more recently, *Medicine in the Medieval Mediterranean* (Bennett 2016 on hospital formularies) and *Textos Médicos – Ediciones Críticas* (Lamagna 2017 on Johannes Actuarius' Greek translation of Avicenna, *De urinis*). See also such volumes as Pritchet 1975 and 1982 (both on Johannes of Alexandria) or Garzya and Masullo 2004 (on Cassius Iatrosophista). To this, one might add editions of *iatrosofia* (for example, Tselikas and Ilioudis 1995 and 1997, or Clark 2011).

since[34], was accompanied by a transformation in the history of science and the history of the book. While the former moved its focus from the *Great Scientists*[35] to the *histoire vécue*[36], the latter shifted from book production[37] to book use, that is, to reading, studying, annotating, sharing, and collecting[38].

Both transformational trends highlighted limitations of Diels' catalogues: they are devoted to authored works with a focus on the major physicians of classical antiquity and of the period that became defined in the meantime as *Late Antiquity*, that is, the period up to the end of the School of Alexandria in the 7th century A.D[39]. With only some exceptions[40], they omit the multiple small, but no less important, anonymous works, notebooks, and other formularies that give witness to the practice of medicine[41], and also many of the physicians of all epochs (but especially the Byzantine ones, also with some exceptions, however[42]) who have not been credited with such a foundational role as Hippocrates and Galen.

---

34 For the proceedings of the first conference, see Garzya 1992. The conference has been fairly consistently held every four years, alternately in Naples and Paris. The many communications presented in each edition dealt with a great many authors and texts, including lesser known physicians and their treatises. The proceedings were first edited by Antonio Garzya, and then by Garzya in collaboration with Jacques Jouanna before being edited by both, along with Véronique Boudon-Millot and Amneris Roselli.

35 As an example of this historiography, see the monumental encyclopedic *Introduction to the History of Science* (1927–1948) of George Sarton (1884–1956).

36 See, for example, Perrin 1988 on the skin (followed by Herida 1998, on skin in the Hippocratic writings), Rey 1993 on pain, or Dumouchel 1995 on emotions. One might also mention here the development of the history of the body, particularly its specific perception and its representation, including its defects (Fischer 1991).

37 The focus on book production might be best identified by the development of codicology, explicitly formalized as a discipline in its own right during this period (see Dain 1949).

38 On this approach, see, for example, the works of Guglielmo Cavallo, particularly Cavallo 1988 about libraries, and Cavallo and Chartier 1995 on reading, with a panoramic presentation of medieval reading culture. On reading Greek medical literature, more specifically, see, for example, Cavallo 1993 or, more recently, Mondrain 2003.

39 On the chonological span of the catalogues (from the 5th century B.C. to the 7th A.D.), see Bruno Rappaport's report in the 1906 issue, p. III.

40 Some of these exceptions might be the *Excerpta* (or *Excerpta varia*) listed for several authors, as well as the pseudepigraphic literature (mostly Hippocratic and Galenic) (see for example the remedies attributed to, or extracted from the works of, Hippocrates [I.48–49] and Galen [I.132–133]), in addition to some *iatrosophia* of the Ottoman period listed mostly under Hippocrates (I.42), Galen (I.123 and N.38) and Meletius (II.64), but also under Erasistratos (II.36) and Magnus (II.59), besides references to *iatrosophic* literature about Iustus (N.56), Logadius (N.56), Lucas (N.56), and Syncellus (N.66).

41 For such works (hospital formularies), see, for example, Bennett, 2016.

42 These exceptions are the following (in alphabetical order of their names as in Diels) with their reference to Diels: Abraham (II.3; N.42), Antonius Pyropulus (II.15; N.45), Beniaminus (II.22;

A *New Diels* is now a desideratum of the scholarly community[43]. While urgently needed, it would require that Greek medical manuscripts be newly catalogued and their texts accurately identified, building on the twentieth-century classical scholarship briefly presented above and indeed, going even further through a renewed *in situ* autoptic analysis of manuscripts and the reading of their many texts[44]. Whereas codicological analysis would allow for a better approximation of the time or period and place of production of the manuscripts (and also of their texts in some cases), reading and precise identification of all their texts would lead to a more complete and accurate knowledge of medical literature and practice from antiquity to the Renaissance, particularly thanks to the treatises of the period posterior to the 7th century and, for all periods, the multiple anonymous texts of all types not considered in Diels' catalogues.

The present work aims to lead the study of Greek medical manuscripts and literature of the classical and post-classical periods in that direction. While it fundamentally reproduces Diels' lists of Greek manuscripts, it reformats them in different, yet complementary, ways and provides new search tools that may be used for at least two purposes: compiling a catalogue of Greek medical manuscripts that will eventually generate the material necessary for a *New Diels*, and investigating the tradition, reception, and intellectual, and scientific history of Greek medical literature and medicine.

N.46), Cassius iatrosophista (II.22; N.46), Chariton (II.23), Constantinus Meliteniota (II.24; N.47), Damascenus (II.25), Eleutherus (II.35), Esdras propheta (II.37–38; N.50–51), Euphemius Siculus (II.38; N.51), Iacobus Psychrestus (II.50), Ioannes Chumnos (II.52), Ioannes Esdra (II.53), Ioannes episcopus Prisdyanesis (II.54; N.55), Ioannes Staphidaces (II.55; N.55), Leo (II.57; N.56), Manuel Comnenus (N.57), Maximus (Planudes?) (II.62; N.57), Neophytus Prodromenus (II.68; N.60), Nicolaus Myrepsus (II.69; N.60), Nicomedes iatrosophista (II.69), Paulus Nicaeensis (II.81; N.63), Perzoe (II.81), Philippus Xerus (N.63), Photius monachus (II.85),Taronitus (II.100; N.67), Theophilus (II.101–106; N.68), Theophylactus Simocata (II.106; N.68), and Ioannes Zacharias Actuarius (II.108–111; N.69).

43 Some *instrumenta studiorum* that might be considered as partial *New Diels* are already available. One of them is the catalogue of the manuscripts of the Latin translations of Hippocrates compiled by Pearl Kibre (above). Other two are the analytical lists of the manuscripts of the Arabic translations of Greek medical literature and original Arabic medical literature compiled by Sezgin 1970 (medicine, pharmacy, and zoology) and 1971 (alchemy, chemistry, botany, and agriculture), and Ullmann 1970 (medicine). One might also add the inventory of illustrated medical manuscripts compiled by MacKinney as early as 1965 (not only Greek and Latin, but also Syriac, Arabic and Turkish, and the roman languages, English, and German). Relevant also, the bibliographical lists compiled by Gerhard Fichtner (1932–2012) for Hippocrates and Galen (first published on demand, with several successive versions from 1985 on, and now available on line on the website of *Corpus Medicorum Graecorum*).

44 For a proposal in that sense, see Touwaide 2018. Whereas a publication upon completion of the research would be highly desirable, a gradual publication of available data in the form of a work in progress on the Internet might be useful, be it for a catalogue of manuscripts or a *New Diels*.

As such, the present work offers a set of new *instrumenta studiorum* for further developments in manuscript studies, the classical, medical and scientific traditions, and medical history.

Each of the five tomes of the present work has a specific content and purpose. The first tome exactly reproduces Diels' lists of Greek medical manuscripts[45], excluding the lists of the manuscripts containing the possible medieval translations of Greek medical texts into Syriac, Arabic, Hebrew, or Latin according to the treatises. It is not a photographic reproduction of Diels' original pages, however. Whereas lists of manuscripts in the original printing of Diels are presented in the form of blocks of continuous texts, they are rearranged here in the form of enumerations that clearly distinguish each item. The bibliography of Diels has been treated in a similar way for the purposes of clarity. The lists of manuscripts and the bibliography comprise most of the first tome, which is complemented by two indices: one of the authors and texts included in Diels, and the other of the manuscripts listed in Diels. For the purposes of easy and direct consultation, both of these indices open the first tome, which aims to not only make Diels available in a handy format, but to facilitate its use in research.

The remaining four tomes differ with regard to substance and purpose. All of them reproduce the contents of the manuscripts as described in Diels, including all annotations about title, *incipit*, *desinit* and lacunae, in addition to possible similarities with other manuscripts, sources, or copies. They proceed by manuscript (instead of by authors and works as in Diels' original publication). Identification of manuscripts exactly reproduces Diels' elements (city, library, and collection as appropriate, followed by shelfmark). The identification of many manuscripts required updating. This is the case for the several items known in Diels through earlier literature without exact identification. It is also the case of the codices destroyed during the two World Wars of the twentieth century, and of those that have changed location after the publication of Diels. Finally, it is also the case for those manuscripts which have received new shelfmarks. For all of these manuscripts, tomes two through five provide supplementary information with their exact identification, their state of preservation and location, or

45 Until a new reprint is published, Diels does not seem to be widely available (in spite of the 1970 reprint). WorldCat lists only 20 copies across the world. Nevertheless, digital copies are available on the Internet with different levels of quality, accuracy, and completeness via such sites as the *Corpus Medicorum Graecorum*, the Royal College of Physicians (RCP) in London, the Medic@ collection of the BIUSanté in Paris, the Digitale Bibliothek of the Münchener DigitalisierungsZentrum of the Bayerische Staatsbibliothek in Munich, and Google. These copies are linked on some other websites such as the Internet Archive, the UK Medical Heritage Library, the Medical Heritage Library, and European Libraries. As mentioned above, a database built on the basis of Diels is available on the website of the Institute for the Preservation of Medical Traditions.

their new shelfmark[46]. Another contribution of these tomes is their index of manuscripts, which includes possible new locations and shelfmarks, thus allowing one to search for manuscripts in two different, yet complementary ways: by their location and shelfmark as in Diels' time or in present time.

Besides these shared features, tomes two through five differ further by their content. Tomes two through four are each devoted to one author or a group of authors: tome two is devoted to Hippocrates, tome three to Galen, and tome four to the authors defined in Diels as *the remaining physicians* (*Die übrigen griechischen Ärzte ausser Galenos und Hippocrates*), that is, all the other authors of classical and late antiquity, with some Byzantine ones as well[47]. These three volumes aim to allow for a general study of the whole manuscript tradition of the textual bodies they are devoted to. Although they still have a limited documentary basis, they compensate for the lack of relevant instruments in currently available literature, and they provide the substance for first reconstructions of the whole tradition of the treatises by (or attributed to) Hippocrates, Galen, and the other Greek physicians considered by Diels.

Tome five goes further in laying down the basis of what will become a general catalogue of Greek medical manuscripts, as it lists the entire contents of all the manuscripts mentioned in Diels. It proceeds as do tomes two through four, by city and library in alphabetical order and, for each library, by collection and shelfmark, with their new locations and identifications as relevant. It also contains all the descriptive annotations about the texts included in Diels. Like tomes two through four, it contains an index of manuscripts that also lists possible new locations and identifications, allowing one to search for manuscripts on the basis of Diels or by their present location and identification.

By reproducing Diels' inventory of, and data on, Greek medical manuscripts, by rearranging them for new investigations, and by providing them with updated identification and new *instrumenta studiorum*, this work aims to not only make Diels newly available in a handy format with updated information and to expand the range of its applications, but to make further strides in the direction of a general catalogue of Greek medical manuscripts. This catalogue, in turn, will lead to the much needed *New Diels* that may be expected to transform the study and understanding of the Greek medical literature and medicine, with their tradition.

46 For these data, see Touwaide, 2016.
47 For these physicians, see note 42.

Bibliography

Ackermann 1791: Johannes Chr. Ackermann, "Caput XXIII De Hippocrate, Medicorum Principe, et Polybo eius Discipulo", in Ioannes Albertus Fabricius, *Bibliotheca Graeca sive Notitia Scriptorum Veterum Graecorum quorumcumque Monumenta Integra aut Fragmenta edita exstant tum plerorumque e MSS. ac deperditis ab auctore recognita*. Editio quarta variorum curis emendatior atque auctior curante Gottlieb Christophoro Harles. Accedunt B. I. A. Fabricii et Christoph. Augusti Heumanni Supplementa inedita, Volumen secundum. Hamburgi: apud Carolum Ernestum Bohn; Lipsiae: Ex Officina Breitkopfia, 1791, pp. 506–611.

Ackermann 1795: Johannes Chr. Ackermann, "Caput III De Dioscoride", in Ioannes Albertus Fabricius, *Bibliotheca Graeca sive Notitia Scriptorum Veterum Graecorum quorumcumque Monumenta Integra aut Fragmenta edita exstant tum plerorumque e MSS. ac deperditis ab auctore recognita*. Editio tertia variorum curis emendatior atque auctior curante Gottlieb Christophoro Harles. Accedunt Christophori Augusti Heumanni Supplementa inedita, Volumen quartum. Hamburgi: apud Carolum Ernestum Bohn; Lipsiae: Ex Officina Breitkopfia et Haertelia, 1795, pp. 673–702.

Ackermann 1796: Johannes Chr. Ackermann, " Caput XIX (olim XVII) Claudius Galenus", in Ioannes Albertus Fabricius, *Bibliotheca Graeca sive Notitia Scriptorum Veterum Graecorum quorumcumque Monumenta Integra aut Fragmenta edita exstant tum plerorumque e MSS. ac deperditis ab auctore recognita*. Editio tertia variorum curis emendatior atque auctior curante Gottlieb Christophoro Harles. Accedunt Christophori Augusti Heumanni Supplementa inedita, Volumen quintum. Hamburgi: apud Carolum Ernestum Bohn; Lipsiae: Ex Officina Breitkopfia et Haertelia, 1796, pp. 377–500.

Ackermann 1821: Johannes Chr. Ackermann, "Historia literaria Claudii Galeni ... ex Jo. Alb. Fabricii Biblioth. Graec. ex ed. Gli. Cph. Harles, vol. V. P. 377–500", in Carolus Gottlob Kühn (ed.), *Claudii Galeni Opera omnia*, Tomus 1 (Medicorum Graecorum Opera quae exstant 1). Leipzig: Carl Cnobloch, 1821, pp. XVII–CCLXV.

Ackermann 1825: Johannes Chr. Ackermann, "Historia literaria Hippocratis ... ex Jo. Alb. Fabricii Biblioth. Graec. ex edit. Gli. Cph. Harles, vol. II. P. 506–511. Desunta et hinc inde aucta et emendata", in Carolus Gottlob Kühn (ed.), *Magni Hippocratis Opera omnia*, Tomus 1 (Medicorum Graecorum Opera quae exstant 21). Leipzig: Carl Cnobloch, 1825, pp. I–CCVI).

Alexanderson 1963: Bengt Alexanderson, *Die Hippokratische Schrift Prognostikon. Überlieferung and Text* (Studia Graeca et Latina Gothoburgensia 17). Göteborg: Acta Universitatis Gothoburgensis, 1963.

Alexanderson 1967: Bengt Alexanderson, *Galenos, Περὶ κρίσεων. Uberlieferung und Text* (Studia Graeca et Latina Gothoburgensia 23). Göteborg: Acta Universitatis Gothoburgensis, 1967.

Bennett 2016: David Bennett, *Medicine and Pharmacy in Byzantine Hospitals. A study of the extant formularies* (Medicine in the Medieval Mediterranean 7). London and New York, NY: Routledge, 2016.

Bersgträsser 1914: Gotthelf Bergsträsser (ed.), *Pseudogaleni in Hippocratis de septimanis* (Corpus Medicorum Graecorum XI 2,1). Lipsiae et Berolini: B.G. Teubner, 1914.

Bernabò 2010: Massimo Bernabò (ed.), *La collezione di testi chirurgici di Niceta. Firenze, Biblioteca Medicea Laurenziana, plut. 74.7. Tradizione medica classica a Bisanzio* (Folia Picta. Manoscritti miniati medievali 2). Roma: Storia e Letteratura, 2010.

Boudon 2000: Véronique Boudon, *Galien*, Tome II: *Exhortation à l'étude de la médecine. Art médical*. Texte établi et traduit (Collection des Universités de France). Paris: Belles Lettres, 2000.

Bouras-Vallianatos 2015: Petros Bouras-Vallianatos, "Greek Manuscripts at the Wellcome Library in London: A Descriptive Catalogue", *Medical History* 59 (2015), pp. 275–326.

Bouras-Vallianatos 2020: Petros Bouras-Vallianatos, "Addenda et Corrigenda to the 'Greek Manuscripts at the Wellcome Library in London: A Descriptive Catalogue', *Medical History* 59 (2015): 275–326", in Petros Bouras-Vallianatos (ed.), *Exploring Greek Manuscripts in the Library at Wellcome Collection in London*. London: Routledge, 2020, pp. 181–182.

Calder et al. 1999: William M. Calder III, and Jaap Mansfeld (eds.), with the participation of Alex Leukart, François Paschould, and Olivier Reverdin, *Hermann Diels (1848–1922) et la science de l'Antiquité. Huit exposés suivis de discussion ... Vandoeuvres-Genève, 17–21 août 1998* (Entretiens sur l'Antiquité classique 45). Genève: Fondation Hardt, 1999.

Cavallo 1988: Guglielmo Cavallo, *Le biblioteche nel mondo antico e medievale* (Biblioteca universale Laterza 250). Bari and Roma: Laterza, 1988.

Cavallo 1993: Guglielmo Cavallo, "Libri di medicina: gli usi di un sapere", in Evelyne Patlagean (ed.), *Maladie et société à Byzance* (Collectanea 3). Spoleto: Centro italiano di studi sull'alto medioevo, 1993, pp. 43–56.

Cavallo and Chartier 1995: Guglielmo Cavallo and Roger Chartier (eds), *Storia della lettura nel mondo occidentale* (Storia e Società). Bari and Roma: Laterza, 1995.

Chatzopoulou 2014: Βενετία Χατζοπούλου, "Δύο ἄγνωστα ἰατρικά χειρόγραφα μὲ ἔργα τοῦ Νικολάου Βελισδονίτη", in Παναγιώτης Βλάχος, *Όσιος Ευγένιος ο Αιτωλός και αι Σχολαί των Αγράφων κατά την Τουρκοκρατία. Καρπενήσιον, 7–9 Όκτωβρίου 2011. Πρακτικά*. Αθήνα: Σύνδεσμος "Ευγένιος ο Αιτωλός", 2014, vol. 2, pp. 573–581.

Clark 2011: Patricia A. Clark, *A Cretan Healer's Handbook in the Byzantine Tradition: Text, Translation and Commentary* (Medicine in the Medieval Mediterranean 3). Aldershot, and Burlington, VT: Ashgate, 2011.

Costomiris 1889: Georges A. Costomiris, "Etudes sur les écrits inédits des anciens médecins grecs et ceux dont le texte original est perdu, mais qui existent en latin ou en arabe. Première série: Hippocrate, Cratevas, Aelius Promotus, Galien", *Revue des études grecques* 1 (1889), pp. 343–383.

Costomiris 1890: Georges A. Costomiris, "Etudes sur les écrits inédits des anciens médecins grecs et ceux dont le texte original est perdu, mais qui existent en latin ou en arabe. Deuxième série: L'Anonyme de Daremberg, Métrodora, Aétius", *Revue des études grecques* 3 (1890), pp. 145–179.

Costomiris 1891: Georges A. Costomiris, "Etudes sur les écrits inédits des anciens médecins grecs et ceux dont le texte original est perdu, mais qui existent en latin ou en arabe. Troisième série: Alexandre (Sophiste et Roi), Timothée, Léon le Sophiste, Théophane Nonnos, les Ephodes", *Revue des études grecques* 4 (1891), pp. 97–110.

Costomiris 1892: Georges A. Costomiris, "Études sur les écrits inédits des anciens médecins grecs. Quatrième série: Hippiatriques et auteurs du XIe siècle: Psellus, Siméon Seth, Damnastès", *Revue des études grecques*, 5 (1892), pp. 61–72.

Costomiris 1897: Georges A. Costomiris, "Etudes sur les écrits inédits des anciens médecins grecs et ceux dont le texte original est perdu, mais qui existent en latin ou en arabe. Cinquième série: XIIIe–XIVe siècles, Jean Tzetzès, Nicolas Myrepsus, Jean Actuarius", *Revue des études grecques* 10 (1897), pp. 405–445.

Dain 1930: Alphonse Dain, *Les manuscrits d'Onesandros* (Collection d'études anciennes). Paris: Belles Lettres, 1930.

Dain 1933: Alphonse Dain, *La tradition du texte d'Héron de Byzance* (Collection d'études anciennes). Paris: Belles Lettres, 1933.

Dain 1946: Alphonse Dain, *Histoire du texte d'Élien le Tacticien des origines à la fin du moyen âge* (Collection d'études anciennes). Paris: Belles Lettres, 1946.

Dain 1949: Alphonse Dain, *Les manuscrits*. Paris: Belles Lettes, 1949.

Daremberg 1845: Charles Daremberg, "Rapport adressé à M. le Ministre de l'Instruction Publique par .. chargé d'une mission médico-littéraire en Allemagne" *Journal général de l'Instruction publique* 14, no. 33 (23 avril 1845), pp. 193–196, and no. 34 (26 avril 1845), pp. 198–202 (also printed as a booklet under the same title, in Paris, P. Dupont, 15 avril 1845, 32 p.).

Daremberg 1848: Charles Daremberg, "Résumé d'un voyage médico-littéraire en Angleterre. Lu à l'Académie des inscriptions et belle-lettres, dans la séance du 6 octobre", *Gazette médicale de Paris*, 4 novembre 1848, pp. 3–18.

Daremberg 1851: Charles Daremberg, "Notices et extraites des manuscrits médicaux d'Angleterre", *Archives des Missions scientifiques et littéraires*, 1851,VII, VIII, and IX.

Daremberg 1852: Charles Daremberg, "Notices et extraites des manuscrits médicaux d'Angleterre", *Archives des Missions scientifiques et littéraires* 1852, I.

Daremberg 1853: Charles Daremberg, *Notices et extraits des manuscrits médicaux grecs, latins et français, des principales bibliothèques de l'Europe, I: Manuscrits grecs d'Angleterre suivis d'un fragment de Gilles de Corbeil et de scolies inédites sur Hippocrate*. Paris: Imprimerie impériale, 1853.

De Boer 1937: Wilko De Boer (ed.), *Galeni De propriorum animi cuiuslibet dignotione et curatione. De animi cuiuslibet peccatorum dignotione et curatione. De atra bile* (Corpus Medicorum Graecorum V 4, 1. 1). Lipsiae et Berolini: B. G. Teubner, 1937.

Dickson 1998: Keith Dickson (ed.), *Stephanus the Philosopher and Physician, Commentary on Galen's Therapeutics to Glaucon* (Studies in Ancient Medicine 19). Leiden, Boston, MA, Köln: Brill, 1998.

Diels 1905: Hermann Diels (ed.), *Die Handschriften der antiken Ärzte. I. Teil. Hippokrates und Galenos. Im Auftrage der akademischen Kommission herausgegeben* (Abhandlungen der Königlich Preussischen Akademie der Wissenschaften vom Jahre 1905, Philosophisch-historische Klasse, Abhandlung III). Berlin: Königliche Akademie der Wissenschaften, 1905.

Diels 1906a: Hermann Diels, *Die Handschriften der antiken Ärzte. II. Teil. Die übrigen griechischen Ärzte ausser Hippokrates und Galenos. Im Auftrage der akademischen Kommission herausgegeben von -* (Abhandlungen der Königlich Preussischen Akademie der Wissenschaften vom Jahre 1906, Philosophisch-historische Klasse, Abhandlung I). Berlin: Königliche Akademie der Wissenschaften, 1906.

Diels 1906b: Hermann Diels, *Die Handschriften der antiken Ärzte. Griechische Abteilung. Im Auftrage der akademischen Kommission herausgegeben von - aus den Abhandlungen der Königlich Preussischen Akademie der Wissenschaften der Jahre 1905 und 1906*. Berlin: Königliche Akademie der Wissenschaften, 1906.

Diels 1908: Hermann Diels, *Bericht über den Stand des interakademischen Corpus Medicorum Antiquorum und Erster Nachtrag zu den in den Abhandlungen 1905 und 1906 veröffentlichten Katalogen: Die Handschriften der antiken Ärzte. I. und II. Teil. Zusammengestellt im Namen der Kommission der Königlich Preussischen Akademie der Wissenschaften von -* (Abhandlungen der Königlich Preussischen Akademie der Wissenschaften vom Jahre 1907, Philosophisch-historische Klasse, Abhandlung II). Berlin: Königliche Akademie der Wissenschaften, 1908.

Diels 1912: Hermann Diels, *Die handschriftliche Überlieferung des galenischen Commentars zum Prorrheticum des Hippocrates* (Abhandlungen der Königlich Preussischen Akademie der Wissenschaften vom Jahre 1912, Philosophisch-historische Klasse, Abhandlung I). Berlin: Königliche Akademie der Wissenschaften, 1912.

Diels et al. 1915: Hermann Diels (ed.), *Galeni, In Hippocratis Prorrheticum I commentaria III*; Johannes Mewaldt (ed.), *Galeni, De comate secundum Hippocratem*; Josef Heeg (ed.), *Galeni, In Hippocratis Prognosticum commentaria III* (Corpus Medicorum Graecorum V 9, 2). Lipsiae et Berolini: B. G. Teubneri, 1915.

Dietz 1832: Friedrich Reinhold Dietz, *Galeni de dissectione musculorum et de consuetudine libri. Ad fidem codicum manuscriptorum alterum secundum, primum alterum graece edidit.* Lipsiae: Leopold Voss, 1832.

Dietz 1834: Friedrich Reinhold Dietz, *Apollonii Citiensis, Stephani, Palladii, Theophili, Meletii, Damasci, Ioannis aliorum Scholia in Hippocratem et Galenum e codicibus mss. Vindobonens. Monacens. Florentin. Mediolanens. Escorialens. etc. primum graece edidit*, 2 volumes. Regimontii Prussorum: apud fratres Borntraeger, 1834.

Dietz 1836: Friedrich Reinhold Dietz, *Severi Iatrosophistae De clysteribus liber. Ad Fidem Codicis Manuscripti unici Florentini primum Graece edidit.* Regimontii Prussorum: apud Fratres Borntraeger, 1836.

Dumouchel 1995: Paul Dumouchel, *Emotions. Essai sur le corps et le social* (Collection Les Empêcheurs de penser en rond). Le Plessis-Robinson: Synthélabo, 1995.

Durling 1967: Richard J. Durling, "Corrigenda and addenda to Diels' Galenica. I. Codices Vaticani". *Traditio* 23 (1967), pp. 461–476.

Durling 1981: Richard J. Durling, "Corrigenda and addenda to Diels' Galenica. II. Codices Miscellanei". *Traditio* 37 (1981), pp. 373–381.

Durling 1985–1993: Richard J. Durling, "A Guide to the Medical Manuscripts Mentioned in Kristeller's *Iter Italicum*", *Traditio* 41 (1985), pp. 341–365; 44 (1988), pp. 485–536; 46 (1991), pp. 347–379; 48 (1993), pp. 253–316.

Eleuteri 1981: Paolo Eleuteri, *Storia della tradizione manoscritta di Museo* (Biblioteca di Studi Antichi 30). Pisa: Giardini, 1981.

Fabricius 1705–1728: Jo. Alberti Fabricii, *Bibliotheca Graeca* ... Hamburgi: Sumptu Christiani Lievezeit, Typis Spiringlanis, 1705–1728, 14 volumes (after the general title as above, each volume has a specific subtitle that details its contents).

Fabricius ed. Harles 1790–1838: Gottlieb Christophorus Harles, *Ioannis Alberti Fabricii ... Bibliotheca Graeca sive notitia scriptorum veterum graecorum quorumcunque monumenta integra aut fragmenta edita exstant tum plerorumque e MSS. ac deperditis ab auctore tertium recognita et plurimis locis aucta editio quarta variorum curis emendatior atque auctior ... Accedunt B. I. A. Fabricii et Christoph. Augusti Heumanni supplementa inedita*. Hamburgi: apud Carolum Ernestum Bohn; Lipsiae: ex Officina Breitkoppia, 1790–1838, 13 volumes.

Fichtner 1985a: Gerhard Fichtner, *Corpus Galenicum. Verzeichnis der galenischen und pseudogalenischen Schriften*. Tübingen: the author, 1985.

Fichtner 1985b: Gerhard Fichtner, *Corpus Hippocraticum. Verzeichnis der hippokratischen und pseudohippokratischen Schriften.* Tübingen: the author, 1985.

Fischer 1991: Jean-Louis Fischer, *Monstres. Histoire du corps et de ses défauts*. Paris: Syros Alternatives, 1991.

Formentin 1978: Mariarosa Formentin, *I codici greci di medicina nelle tre Venezie* (Università di Padova, Studi bizantini e neogreci 10). Padova: Liviana editrice, 1978.

Formentin 1997: Maria Rosa Formentin, "Codici greci di medicina nella Biblioteca Nazionale Vittorio Emanuele III di Napoli: le vie di acquisizione", in Sergio Sconocchia and Lucio Toneatto (eds.), in collaboration with Daria Crismani, Michele Faraguna, and Italo Pin, *Lingue tecniche del greco e del latino II. Atti del II Seminario internazionale sulla letteratura scientifica e tecnica greca e latina (Trieste, 4–5 ottobre 1993)*. Bologna: Pàtron, 1997, pp. 208–216.

Fortuna and Raia 2006: Stefania Fortuna and Annamaria Raia, "Corrigenda and Addenda to Diels *Galenica* by Richard J. Durling: III. Manuscripts and Editions", *Traditio* 61 (2006), pp. 1–30.

Garzya 1992: Antonio Garzya (ed.), *Tradizione e ecdotica dei testi medici tardo-antichi e bizantini. Atti del Convegno internazionale, Anacapri, 29–31 ottobre 1990* (Collectanea 5). Napoli: D'Auria, 1992.

Garzya and Masullo 2004: Antonio Garzya and Rita Masullo (eds), *I problemi di Cassio Iatrosofista. Testo critico, introduzione, apparato critico, traduzione e note*. Napoli: Accademia Pontaniana, 2004.

Green 1996: Monica H. Green, "A Handlist of the Latin and Vernacular Manuscripts of the So-Called Trotula Texts. Part I: The Latin Manuscripts", *Scriptorium* 50 (1996), pp. 137–175.

Green 1997: Monica H. Green, "A Handlist of the Latin and Vernacular Manuscripts of the So-Called Trotula Texts. Part II: The Vernacular Texts and Latin Re-Writings", *Scriptorium* 51 (1997), pp. 80–104.

Haller 1771–1772: Albrecht von Haller, *Bibliotheca botanica qua scripta ad rem herbariam facientia a rerum initiis recensentur*, 2 volumes. Tiguri: Orell, Gessner, Fuessli, et Socc., 1771–1772.

Haller 1774–1775: Albrecht von Haller, *Bibliotheca chirurgica qua scripta ad artem chirurgicam facientia a rerum initiis recensentur*, 2 volumes. Bernae: Em. Haller; Basileae: Joh. Schweighauser, 1774–1775.

Haller 1774–1777: Albrecht von Haller, *Bibliotheca anatomica qua scripta ad anatomen et physiologiam facientia a rerum initiis recensentur*, 2 volumes. Tiguri: Orell, Gessner, Fuessli, et Socc., 1774–1777.

Haller 1776–1788: Albrecht von Haller, *Bibliotheca medicinae practicae qua scripta ad partem medicinae practicam facientia a rerum initiis ad A. MDCCLXXV recensentur*, 4 volumes. Basileae: Joh. Schweighauser, and Bernae: Em. Haller, 1776–1788.

Heiberg 1921–1924: Johannes L. Heiberg (ed.), *Paulus Aegineta*, 2 volumes (Corpus Medicorum Graecorum IX 1–2). Lipsiae et Berolini: B. G. Teubner, 1921–1924.

Heiberg et al. 1927: Johannes L. Heiberg, Johannes Mewaldt, Ernst Nachmanson, Hermann Schoene (eds), *Hippocratis opera: Indices librorum, Iusiurandum, Lex, De arte, De medico, De decente habitu, Praeceptiones, De prisca medicina, De aere locis aquis, De alimento, De liquidorum usu, De flatibus* (Corpus Medicorum Graecorum I 1). Lipsiae et Berolini: B. G. Teubner, 1927.

Helmreich 1913: Georg Helmreich, *Handschriftliche Studien zu Symeon Seth* (Programm des K. humanistischen Gymnasiums in Ansbach für das Schuljahr 1912/13). Ansbach: C. Brügel & Sohn, 1913.

Henry 1938: Paul Henry, *Études Plotiniennes I. Les Etats du texte de Plotin* (Museum Lessianum, Section Philosophique, no 20). Paris: Desclée de Brouwer et Cie; Bruxelles: L'Edition Universelle, 1938.

Henry 1941: Paul Henry, *Études Plotiniennes II. Les Manuscrits des Ennéades* (Museum Lessianum, Section Philosophique 21). Bruxelles: L'Edition Universelle; Paris: Desclée de Brouwer et Cie, and A. et J. Picard, 1941.

Herida 1998: Magid Herida, *La peau dans les écrits hippocratiques* (Thèse de médecine). Paris: Université Paris 6, 1998.

Hunger and Kresten 1969: Herbert Hunger, and Otto Kresten, *Katalog der griechischen Handschriften der Österreichischen Nationalbibliothek*, Teil 2: *Codices juridici, codices medici* (Museion, Veröffentlichungen der Österreichischen Nationalbibliothek, Neue Folge, Vierte Reihe: Veröffentlichungen der Handschriftensammlung, Erster Band: Katalog der griechischen Handschriften der Österreichischen Nationalbibliothek, Teil 2). Wien: Georg Prachner, 1969.

Ieraci Bio 1989: Anna Maria Ieraci Bio, "La trasmissione della letteratura medica greca nell'Italia meridionale fra X e XV secolo", in Antonio Garzya (ed.), *Contributi alla cultura greca nell'Italia meridionale* (Hellenica et Byzantina Neapolitana 13). Napoli: Bibliopolis, 1989, pp. 133–257.

Ihm 2002: Sibylle Ihm, *Clavis Commentariorum der antiken medizinischen Texte* (Clavis Commentariorum Antiquitatis et Medii Aevi 1). Leiden, Boston and Köln: Brill, 2002.

Ilberg 1911: Johannes Ilberg, *Die Überlieferung der Gynäkologie des Soranos von Ephesos* (Abhandlungen der philologisch-historischen Klasse der Königl. Sächsischen Gesellschaft der Wissenschaften Bd. 28, Abhandlung 2). Leipzig: B. G. Teubner, 1911.

Ilberg 1927: Ioannes Ilberg (ed.), *Soranus* (Corpus Medicorum Graecorum IV). Lipsiae et Berolini: B. G. Teubner, 1927.

Irigoin 1952: Jean Irigoin, *Histoire du Texte de Pindare* (Etudes et Commentaires 13). Paris: Klincksieck, 1952.

Irigoin 1970: Jean Irigoin, "Les manuscrits grecs. I. Quelques catalogues récents", *Revue des études grecques* 83 (1970), pp. 500–529.

Joly 1978: Robert Joly, *Hippocrate. Oeuvres complètes*, Tome XIII: *Les lieux dans l'homme. Du système des glandes. Des fistules. Des hémorrhoïdes. De la vision. Des chairs. De la dentition*. Texte établi et traduit (Collection des Universités de France). Paris: Belles Lettres, 1978.

Karas 1994: Γιάννης Καράς, *Οι επιστήμες στην Τουρκοκρατία. Χειρόγραφα και έντυπα*, Τόμος Γ': Οι επιστήμες της ζώης. Παράρτημα. Έργα γενικόν γνωσέων (Κέντρο Νεοελληνικών Ερευνών, Έθνικό Ίδρυμα Ερευνών 48). Αθήνα: Βιβλιοπωλείον της «Εστίας», 1994.

Kibre 1975–1982: Pearl Kibre, "Hippocrates Latinus. Repertorium of Hippocratic Writings in the Latin Middle Ages", *Traditio* 31 (1975), pp. 99–126; 32 (1976), pp. 257–292; 33 (1977), pp. 253–295; 34 (1978), pp. 193–226; 35 (1979), pp. 273–302; 36 (1980), pp. 347–392; 37 (1981), pp. 267–289; 38 (1982), pp. 165–192.

Kibre 1985: Pearl Kibre, *Hippocrates Latinus. Repertorium of Hippocratic Writings in the Latin Middle Ages*. Revised Edition. New York: Fordham University Press, 1985.

Koch et al. 1923: Konrad Koch (ed.), *Galeni, De sanitate tuenda libri VI*; Georg Helmreich (ed.), *Galeni, De alimentorum facultatibus libri III*; *Galeni, De bonis malisque sucis lber*; Karl Kalbfleisch (ed.), *Galeni, De victu attenuante*; Otto Hartlich (ed.), *Galeni, De ptisana* (Corpus Medicorum Graecorum V 4, 2). Lipsiae et Berolini: B. G. Teubner, 1923.

Kollesch 1973: Jutta Kollesch, "Hermann Diels in seiner Bedeutung für die Geschichte der antiken Medizin", *Philologus* 117 (1973), pp. 278–283.

Kollesch 1989: "Die Erschliessung der antiken medizinischen Texte und ihre Probleme – das *Corpus Medicorum Graecorum et Latinorum*", *Gesnerus* 46 (1989), pp. 195–210.

Kollesch 1999: "Die Organisation und Herausgabe des *Corpus Medicorum Graecorum*: ergänzenden Details aus der Korrespondenz zwischen Hermann Diels und Johannes Mewaldt", in William M. Calder III, and Jaap Mansfeld (eds.), with the participation of Alex Leukart, François Paschould, and Olivier Reverdin, *Hermann Diels (1848–1922) et la science de l'Antiquité. Huit exposés suivis de discussion ... Vandoeuvres-Genève, 17–21 août 1998* (Entretiens sur l'Antiquité classique 45). Genève: Fondation Hardt, 1999, pp. 207–223.

Kudlien 1960: Fridolf Kudlien, *Die handschriftliche Überlieferung des Galenkommentars zu Hippokrates de articulis* (Deutsche Akademie der Wissenschaften zu Berlin, Schriften der Sektion für Altertumswissenschaft 27). Berlin: Akademie Verlag, 1960.

Kudlien 1970: Fridolf Kudlien (ed.), *Hermann Alexander Diels, Die Handschriften der antiken Ärzte. I Hippokrates und Galenos II Die übrigen griechische Ärzte III Nachtrag*. Mit einem Vorwort. Leipzig: Zentralantiquariat der deutschen demokratischen Republik, 1970.

Kühn 1821: Karl Gottlieb Kühn (ed.), *Claudii Galeni Opera omnia*, Tomus I (Medicorum graecorum opera quae exstant 1). Lipsiae: Cnobloch, 1821.

Kühn 1825: Karl Gottlieb Kühn (ed.), *Magni Hippocratis Opera omnia*, Tomus I (Medicorum graecorum opera quae exstant 21). Lipsiae: Cnobloch, 1825.

Lamagna 2017: Mario Lamagna, *Giovanni Attuario, L'eccellente trattato sulle urine di Avicenna*. Introduzione, testo critico, traduzione e note al testo (Serie Textos Médicos – Ediciones Críticas.

Ediciones críticas de la Escuela de traductores de Toledo 21). Cuenca: Ediciones de la Universidad de Castilla-La Mancha, 2017.

MacKinney 1965: Loren MacKinney, *Medical Illustrations in Medieval Manuscripts* (Publications of the Wellcome Historical Medical Library, New Series, V). London: Wellcome Historical Medical Library, 1965.

Marx 1915: Fridericus Marx (ed.), *A. Cornelii Celsi quae supersunt* (Corpus Medicorum Latinorum I). Lipsiae et Berolini: In aedibus B. G. Teubneri, 1915.

Masullo 2006: Rita Masullo, "Sul ΠΕΡΙ ΣΦΥΓΜΩΝ attribuito a Mercurio Monaco", in Véronique Boudon-Millot, Antonio Garzya, Jacques Jouanna, and Amneris Roselli (eds.), *Ecdotica e ricezione dei testi medici greci. Atti del V Convegno Internazionale Napoli, 1–2 ottobre 2004* (Collectanea 24). Napoli: M. D'Auria, 2006, pp. 335–346.

Mewaldt et al. 1914: Johannes Mewaldt (ed.), *Galeni, In Hippocratis De natura hominis commentaria III*; Georg Helmreich (ed.), *Galeni, In Hippocratis De victu acutorum commentaria IV*; Johann Westenberger (ed.), *Galeni, De diaeta Hippocratis in morbis acutis* (Corpus Medicorum Graecorum V 9, 1). Lipsiae et Berolini: B. G. Teubner, 1914.

Mercati 1916: Giovanni Mercati, "Minuzie. – 6–8. Pretesi scritti di Paolo l'Egineta e di Galeno. – 9–11. Pretesi scritti di medicina greca", *Bessarione* 32 (1916), pp. 208–211 (reprinted in Giovanni Mercati, *Opere minori raccolte in occasione del settantesimo natalizio sotto gli auspicii di S. S. Pio XI*, vol. 3 [1907–1916] (Studi e Testi 780. Città del Vaticano: Biblioteca Apostolica Vaticana, 1937, pp. 521–524).

Mercati 1917a: Giovanni Mercati, "Minuzie. – 13–17. Altre correzioni ed aggiunte all'op. Die Handschriften der antiken Aerzte. – 18. Per Aezio", *Bessarione* 38 (1917), pp. 50–55 (reprinted in Giovanni Mercati, *Opere minori raccolte in occasione del settantesimo natalizio sotto gli auspicii di S. S. Pio XI*, vol. 4 [1917–1936] (Studi e Testi 79). Città del Vaticano: Biblioteca Apostolica Vaticana, 1937, pp. 16–21).

Mercati 1917b: Giovanni Mercati, "I. Filippo Xeros Reggino, Giovanni Alessandrino iatrosofista e altri nel codice Vaticano degli Ephodia, and II. Un nuovo capitolo di Sorano e tre nuove ricette superstiziose in Aezio", in Giovanni Mercati, *Notizie varie di antica letteratura medica e di bibliografia* (Studi e Testi 31). Roma: Tipografia Poliglotta Vaticana, 1917, pp. 9–41, and 42–46.

Mondrain 2003: Brigitte Mondrain, "Comment était lu Galien à Byzance dans la première moitié du XVe siècle? Contribution à quelques aspects de l'histoire des textes", in Antonio Garzya and Jacques Jouanna (eds), *Trasmissione e ecdotica dei testi medici greci. Atti del IV Convegno internazionale, Parigi 17–19 maggio 2001* (Collectanea 21). Napoli: D'Auria, 2003, pp. 361–384.

Morani 1981: Moreno Morani, *La tradizione manoscritta del "De natura hominis" di Nemesio* (Scienze filologiche e letteratura 18). Milano: Vita e pensiero, 1981.

Nutton 2004: Vivian Nutton, "Ancient Medicine: From Berlin to Baltimore", in Frank Huisman, and John Harley Warner (eds), *Locating Medical History. The Stories and Their Meanings.* Baltimore, MD, and London: Johns Hopkins University Press, 2004, pp. 115–138.

Olivier 1995: Jean-Marie Olivier, *Répertoire des bibliothèques et des catalogues de manuscrits grecs de Marcel Richard. Troisième édition entièrement refondue* (Corpus Christianorum). Turnhout: Brepols, 1995.

Olivier 2018: Jean-Marie Olivier, *Supplément au répertoire des bibliothèques et des catalogues de manuscrits grecs,* 2 volumes (Corpus Christianorum). Turnhout: Brepols, 2018.

Olivieri 1935: Alessandro Olivieri (ed.), *Aetii Amideni Libri medicinales I–IV* (Corpus Medicorum Graecorum VIII 1). Lipsiae et Berolini: B. G. Teubner, 1935.

***Paléographie* 1977:** *La paléographie grecque et byzantine: actes du colloque international sur la paléographie grecque et byzantine organisé dans le cadre des colloques internationaux du Centre*

National de la recherche scientifique, Paris du 21 au 25 octobre 1974 (Issue 559 of Colloques internationaux du Centre National de la Recherche Scientifique 559). Paris: Editions du CNRS, 1977.

Perilli 1999: Lorenzo Perilli, "La tradizione manoscritta del Glossario ippocratico di Galeno (e l'ordinamento alfabetico delle glosse)", in Antonio Garzya, and Jacques Jouanna (eds.), *I testi medici greci. Tradizione e ecdotica. Atti del III Convegno Internazionale, Napoli 15–18 ottobre 1997.* Napoli: M. D'Auria, 1999, pp. 429–456.

Perilli 2011: Lorenzo Perilli, "Nuovi manoscritti del Glossario Ippocratico di Galeno e considerazioni stemmatiche. *Codex olim Mosquensis, codex Bodleianus Holkhamensis 92*", in Lorenzo Perilli, Christian Brockmann, Klaus-Dietrich Fischer, and Amneris Roselli (eds), *Officina Hippocratica. Beiträge zu Ehren von Anargyros Anastassiou und Dieter Irmer* (Beiträge zur Altertumskunde 289). Berlin and Boston, MA: De Gruyter, 2011, pp. 177–201.

Perrin 1988: Christophe Perrin, *La peau ou la représentation du corps malade: médecines antiques, médecine anatomo-clinique* (Thèse médecine) Nice: Université de Nice, 1988.

Petit 2006: Caroline Petit, "Les manuscrits de Modène et la tradition de l'*Introductio sive medicus* du Pseudo-Galien", in Véronique Boudon-Millot, Antonio Garzya, Jacques Jouanna, and Amneris Roselli (eds), *Ecdotica e ricezione dei testi medici greci. Atti del V Convegno Internazionale, Napoli, 1–2 ottobre 2004* (Collectanea 24). Napoli: M. D'Auria, 2006, pp. 167–185.

Pietrobelli 2010: Antoine Pietrobelli, "Variation autour du Thessalonicensis Vlatadon 14: un manuscrit copié au Xénon du Kral, peu avant la chute de Constantinople", *Revue des études byzantines* 68 (2010), pp. 95–126.

Pritchet 1975: Christopher Dixon Pritchet (ed.), *Iohannis Alexandrini Commentaria in sextum librum Hippocratis Epidemiarum recognovit et adnotatione critica instruxit.* Leiden: Brill, 1975.

Pritchet 1982: Christopher Dixon Pritchet (ed.), *Iohannis Alexandrini Commentaria in librum De sectis Galeni.* Recognovit et adnotatione critica instruxit. Leiden: E. J. Brill, 1982.

Raeder 1926: Ioannes Raeder (ed.), *Oribasii, Synopsis ad Eustathium; Libri ad Eunapium* (Corpus Medicorum Graecorum VI 3). Lipsiae et Berolini: B. G. Teubner, 1926.

Raeder 1928–1933: Ioannes Raeder (ed.), *Oribasii, Collectionum medicarum reliquiae*, 4 volumes (Corpus Medicorum Graecorum VI 1, 1–2; VI 2, 1–2). Lipsiae et Berolini: B. G. Teubner, 1928–1933.

Regling 1920: Kurt Regling, "Bruno Rappaport. Geb. den 4. November 1875, gest. den 20. Juli 1915", *Biographisches Jahrbuch für die Altertumswissenschaft* 40 (1920), pp. 76–83.

Rey 1993: Roselyne Rey, *Histoire de la douleur* (Histoire des sciences). Paris: La Découverte, 1993.

Richard 1948: Marcel Richard, *Répertoire des bibliothèques et des catalogues de nanuscrits grecs* (Publications de l'Institut de recherche et d'histoire des textes 1). Paris: Centre de documentation du Centre National de la Recherche Scientifique, 1948.

Richard 1958: Marcel Richard, *Répertoire des bibliothèques et des catalogues de manuscrits grecs.* Deuxième édition (Centre national de la recherche scientifique, Publications de l'Institut de recherche et d'histoire des textes 1). Paris: Centre national de la recherche scientifique, 1958.

Richard 1964: Marcel Richard, *Répertoire des bibliothèques et des catalogues de manuscrits grecs. Supplément I (1958–1963)* (Documents, études et répertoires publiés par l'Institut de recherche et d'histoire des textes 9). Paris: Éditions du Centre National de la Recherche Scientifique, 1964.

Rivier 1962: André Rivier, *Recherches sur la tradition manuscrite du traité hippocratique "De morbo sacro"* (Travaux publiés sous les auspices de la Société suisse des sciences morales 3). Berne: Francke, 1962.

Roselli 2009: Amneris Roselli, "Due manoscritti medici greci nelle biblioteche di Sofia", *Galenos* 3 (2009), pp. 177–180.

Sarton 1927–1948: George Sarton, *Introduction to the History of Science*, 3 volumes in five tomes. Baltimore: Williams & Wilkins, 1927–1948.

Sezgin 1970: Fuat Sezgin, *Geschichte des arabischen Schrifttums*, Band 3: *Medizin, Pharmazie, Zoologie, Tierheilkunde bis ca. 430 H.* Leiden: E.J.Brill, 1970.

Sezgin 1971: Fuat Sezgin, *Geschichte des arabischen Schrifttums*, Band 4: *Alchimie, Chemie, Botanik, Agrikultur bis ca. 430 H.* Leiden: E.J.Brill, 1971.

Sinkewicz 1990: Robert E. Sinkewicz, *Manuscript Listings for the Authors of Classical and Late Antiquity* (Greek Index Project Series 3). Toronto: Pontifical Institute of Mediaeval Studies, 1990.

Sinkewicz 1992: Robert E. Sinkewicz, *Manuscript Listings for the Authors of the Patristic and Byzantine Periods* (Greek Index Project Series 4). Toronto: Pontifical Institute of Mediaeval Studies, 1992.

Sinkewicz and Hayes 1989: Robert E. Sinkewicz and Walter H. Hayes, *Manuscript Listings for the Authored Works of the Palaeologan Period* (Greek Index Project Series 2). Toronto: Pontifical Institute of Mediaeval Studies, 1989.

Sonderkamp 1987: Joseph A. M. Sonderkamp, *Untersuchung zur Überlieferung der Schriften des Theophanes Chrysobalantes (sog. Theophanes Nonnus)* (Freie Universität Berlin, Byzantinisch–Neogriechisches Seminar, ΠΟΙΚΙΛΑ ΒΥΖΑΝΤΙΝΑ 7). Bonn: Dr. Rudolf Habelt, 1987.

Sprengel 1829: Kurt Sprengel (ed.), *Pedanii Dioscoridis Anazarbei De materia medica ad fidem codicum manuscriptorum, editionis aldinae principis usquequaque neglectae, et interpretum priscroum textum recnesuit, varias addidit lectiones, interpretationem emendavit, commentario illustravit*, Tomus I (Medicorum graecorum opoera quae exstant 1). Lipsiae: Cnobloch, 1829.

Thorndike and Kibre 1937: Lynn Thorndike, and Pearl Kibre, *A Catalogue of Incipits of Mediaeval Scientific Writings in Latin* (Mediaeval Academy of America, Publication 29). Cambridge, MA: Mediaeval Academy of America, 1937.

Thorndike and Kibre 1963: Lynn Thorndike, and Pearl Kibre, *A Catalogue of Incipits of Mediaeval Scientific Writings in Latin*. Revised and augmented edition (Mediaeval Academy of America, Publication 29). Cambridge, MA: Mediaeval Academy of America, 1963.

Touwaide 2009: Alain Touwaide, "Byzantine Medical Manuscripts. Towards a New Catalogue, with a Specimen for an Annotated Checklist of Manuscripts based on an Index of Diels' Catalogue", *Byzantion* 79 (2009), pp. 453–595.

Touwaide 2010: Alain Touwaide, "Codicology and Paleography", in Albrecht Classen (ed.), *Handbook of Medieval Studies. Terms, Methods, Trends*, 3 volumes. Berlin and New York, NY: Walter de Gruyter, 2010, vol. 1, pp. 266–329.

Touwaide 2016: Alain Touwaide, *A Census of Greek Medical Manuscripts. From Byzantium to the Renaissance* (Medicine in the Medieval Mediterranean 6). London and New York, NY: Routledge, 2016.

Touwaide 2018: Alain Touwaide, "Towards a Catalogue of Greek Medical Manuscripts", in Paola Degni, Paolo Eleuteri, and Marilena Maniaci (eds), *Greek Manuscript Cataloguing: Past, Present, and Future* (Bibliologia. Elementa ad librorum studia pertinentia 47). Turnhout: Brepols, 2018, pp. 111–118.

Tselikas 1995: Ἀγαμέμνων Τσελίκας, "Τὰ ἑλληνικὰ γιατροσόφια: μιὰ περιφρονημένη κατηγορία χειρογράφων", in Thanasis Diamantopoulos (ed.), Ιατρικά Βυζάντινα χειρόγραφα. Αθήνα: Δόμος, 1995, pp. 57–69.

Tselikas 2014: Ἀγαμέμνων Τσελίκας, "Δύο συναγωγὲς ἰατρικῶν λέξεων καὶ ἰατρικὲς συνταγὲς ἀπὸ τὸν ἰατροσοφικὸ κώδικα Παναγίου Τάφου 339 τοῦ Πατριαρχείου Ἱρουσολύμων", in *Εύκρατον- Πρακτικά Επιστημονικής Συνάντησης προς τιμήν του κ. Γεωργίου Ν. Αντονακοπούλου ομότιμου καθηγητού της Ιατρικής Σχολής του Πανεπιστημίου Θεσσαλίας. Λάρισσα 10 Μαΐου 2014, Αμφι-*

θέατρο Δημοσίας Κεντρικής Βιβλιοθήκης Λάρισσας «Κωνσταντίνος Κούμας». Λάρισσα: Δημοσίας Κεντρικής Βιβλιοθήκης Λάρισσας «Κωνσταντίνος Κούμας» – Ιατρική Σχολή Πανεπιστημίου Θεσσαλίας, 2014, pp. 107–176.

Tselikas and Ilioudis 1995: Ἀγαμέμνων Τσελίκας, Γιάννης Ἠλιούδης, *Νικολάου Ἱερόπαιδος ἐξ Ἀγράφων, Πραγματεία περὶ Φυσιολογίας καὶ Παθολογίας* (Βιβλιοθήκη Νεωτέρων Ἑλληνῶν Ἰατρῶν 1). Λάρισα: Πανεπιστήμιο Θεσσαλίας, Τμῆμα Ἰατρικῆς, 1995.

Tselikas and Ilioudis 1997: Ἀγαμέμνων Τσελίκας, Γιάννης Ἠλιούδης, *Νικολάου Ἱερόπαιδος ἐξ Ἀγράφων, Ἐκδόσεις μερικαὶ εἰς ἀρχάριον ἰατρόν* (Βιβλιοθήκη Νεωτέρων Ἑλληνῶν Ἰατρῶν 2). Λάρισα: Πανεπιστήμιο Θεσσαλίας, Τμῆμα Ἰατρικῆς, 1997.

Turyn 1932: Aleksander Turyn, *De Codicibus Pindaricis* (Polska Akademja Umiejętności: Archiwum Filologiczne 11). Cracoviae: Academia Polonae Litterarum, 1932.

Turyn 1943: Aleksander Turyn, *The Manuscript Tradition of the Tragedies of Aeschylus*. New York, NY: Polish Institute of Arts and Sciences in America, 1943.

Turyn 1952: Alexander Turyn, *Studies in the Manuscript Tradition of the Tragedies of Sophocles* (Illinois Studies in Language and Literature 36, 1–2.). Urbana, IL: University of Illinois Press, 1952.

Turyn 1957: Alexander Turyn, *The Byzantine Manuscript Tradition of the Tragedies of Euripides* (Illinois Studies in Language and Literature 43). Urbana, IL: University of Illinois Press, 1957.

Ullmann 1970: Manfred Ullmann, *Die Medizin im Islam* (Handbuch der Orientalistik, Erste Abteilung: Der nahe und der mittlere Osten, Ergänzungsband VI, 1. Abschnitt). Leiden and Köln: Brill, 1970.

Verner 1966: Mathilde Verner "Johann Albert Fabricius, Eighteenth-Century Scholar and Bibliographer", *The Papers of the Bibliographical Society of America* 60 (3) (1966), pp. 281–326.

Voigts and Kurtz 2004: Linda Ersham Voigts, and Patricia Deery Kurtz, *Electronic Thorndike Kibre (eTK) and Electronic Voigts Kurtz (eVK)*. CD Rom publication, release 20 August 2004.

Vollmer 1916: Fridericus Vollmer, *Quinti Sereni Liber medicinalis*. Edidit – (Corpus Medicorum Latinorum II 3). Lipsiae et Berolini: B. G. Teubner, 1916.

Wellmann 1908: Max Wellmann (ed.), *Philumeni de venenatis animalibus eorumque remediis ex codice vaticano* primum edidit (Corpus Medicorum Graecorum X 1, 1). Lipsiae et Berolini: B. G. Teubner, 1908.

Wenkebach 1934: Ernst Wenkebach (ed.), *Galeni, In Hippocratis epidemiarum librum I commentarii III*; Franz Pfarr (Germ. transl.), *Galeni, In Hippocratis epidemiarum librum II commentarii V* (Corpus Medicorum Graecorum V 10, 1). Lipsiae et Berolini: B. G. Teubner, 1934.

Wenkebach 1936: Ernst Wenkebach (ed.), *Galeni, In Hippocratis epidemiarum librum IIII commentarii III* (Corpus Medicorum Graecorum V 10, 2. 1). Lipsiae et Berolini: B. G. Teubner, 1936.

Wilson 1987: Nigel G. Wilson, "Aspects of the Transmission of Galen", in Guglielmo Cavallo (ed.), *Le strade del testo* (Studi e commenti 5). Bari: Adriatica Editrice, 1987, pp. 45–64.

Zipser 2009: Barbara Zipser (ed.), *John the Physician's Therapeutics. A Medical Handbook in Vernacular Greek* (Studies in Ancient Medicine 37). Leiden: Brill, 2009.

Acknowledgements

This work is the result of decades of intensive activity in libraries, research centers, universities, and other institutions throughout the world, which have all provided resources, access to collections, expertise and guidance and, most simply, a home. I am pleased to thank all of them and their staff, even though I cannot enumerate them here. In very recent years, the work has benefitted from the active support of De Gruyter, particularly the Senior Editor for Classical Studies Dr. Serena Pirrotta and her team, especially Marco Acquafredda, and De Gruyter computer and technical units in the persons of Anne Hiller and Florian Ruppenstein who have provided much needed assistance. Going slightly back in time, Patricia Kellogg has been an efficient research assistant and Cheyenne Moore has checked the accuracy of my index of Diels against the original. Since its foundation in 2007 the *Institute for the Preservation of Medical Traditions* has hosted the programme. In the very last phase, Marisa Gomez has checked with great linguistic talent the correctness of the introduction to the several parts of the work. More than anyone else, Emanuela Appetiti has accompanied me through multiple peregrinations of all kinds of which this work may give only an imperfect idea. I cannot conclude without remembering Joseph A. M. Sonderkamp with whom I discussed the project of a *New Diels* and a catalogue of Greek medical manuscripts as early as 1983 in Berlin and then in 1987 at Louvain-la-Neuve. We had defined a cooperative programme and had started implementing it when the sinister *Moira* decided shortly after that we would not fully realize it in collaboration.

Index of Manuscripts
Diels' Location and Shelfmark

Notes for consultation

This index lists all the manuscripts with Galenic texts mentioned in Diels. The identifications exactly reproduce the data provided in Diels, the majority of which comprise the following three or four components: city (German form), library (mostly in the original language, often in an abbreviated form, and in their form as in Diels' time), collection (when appropriate), and one or more shelfmarks or references to an earlier work. In some cases, the name of the library is not explicitly mentioned; it can be identified through the list of catalogues in Diels' bibliography. The index references the page number(s) where each item appears in the present volume.

This index is preceded by a **Finding Aid** which lists the city, library and collection names in alphabetical order with reference to the present index, and two lists: one with the names as in Diels (sometimes including transliteration into the Latin alphabet for Greek names) and the other with their current standard English form.

Finding Aid
City and Library names

1. Names according to Diels

2. Standard English names

Index of Manuscripts

Index of Manuscripts
Current location and shelfmark

Notes for consultation

This index lists all the Greek manuscripts with Galenic texts mentioned in Diels that have been preserved and identified since[1]. Their designation comprises their current location and shelfmark, with the following three or four components: city, library, collection (when appropriate), and shelfmark. All names are in the original language and alphabet, followed by their transliteration into Latin alphabet and translation into English for those in the original Russian and Armenian alphabet and form. Each entry of the index references the page number(s) in this volume where the manuscripts appear.

Since the manuscripts contained in the catalogue in this volume are identified as they are in Diels, consultation of the catalogue on the basis of this index might be problematic because current designations do not always match Diels' designations. In Diels, indeed, cities are identified by their German names, libraries are often designated in an abbreviated form, collection names are abbreviated or may not reflect actual names, and shelfmarks are sometimes insufficient or inexact, or even include earlier ones. Additionally, changes have occurred since Diels' time in the location of some collections and several manuscripts, in the names of some libraries and, also, in the shelfmarks (and even in the shelfmark system) of several libraries. Diels' identifiers are reproduced between parentheses after the page number referring to the mention(s) of the manuscripts in the catalogue contained in this volume. In the catalogue itself, both designations of manuscripts are included when appropriate, followed by the current one (as listed in the present index).

This index is preceded by a **Finding Aid** which provides the current city, library, and collection names in alphabetical order with reference to the present index. All names are in the original language and alphabet.

---

1 This index does not include the manuscripts that have been lost or destroyed (*in toto* or *in parte*) since (e.g. some items from Dresden or Torino), the manuscripts that cannot be exactly identified on the basis of Diels' information, the papyri, and the Latin and Arabic manuscripts included among the Greek manuscripts in Diels. The identifications reproduce those in Touwaide 2016.

Finding Aid

City and Library names

[2] Actually Μοναστική Πολιτεία Αγίου Όρους.

Index of Manuscripts

Bologna, Biblioteca Universitaria
1808: 12
2678 (1678 [ol. 228]): 12
3632: 12
3636: 13
3637: 13

Bruxelles, Bibliothèque royale de Belgique
See Brüssel, Königl. Bibl.
11345–48: 13

Cambridge, Gonville and Caius College
See Cambridge, Caius Coll.
47/24: 14 (47), [946], 15 ([6605])
76/43: 14 (76), 15 ([949])
355/582: 14 (355), 15 ([948])
360/587: 14 (360)

Cambridge, University Library
See Cambridge, Cantabrig., Bibl. Univ.
Ff. 3. 30: 15 (F. F. 3. 30)

Carpentras, Bibliothèque municipale Inguimbertine
See Carpentras, Bibl. Inguimbertine
Ms 1774: 15 (nr. 1774 [P., V])

Città del Vaticano, Biblioteca Apostolica Vaticana
See Rom, Bibl. Vaticana
Archivio di San Pietro
H 45: 89 (Rom, Bibl. St. Petri H 45)
Barberiniani
See Rom, Bibl. Barberin.
5: 88 (I 5)
80: 88 (I 80 [273])
118: 88 (I 118)
127: 88 (I 127)
152: 88 (I 152)
344: 89 (III 63 [= 245])
Ottoboniani
311: 90

Genève, Bibliothèque de Genève
MS grec 42: 27 (Genf, Genev. Bibl. Urb. 42)

Grottaferrata, Biblioteca del Monumento nazionale di Grottaferrata
Z.γ.VI (GR 81): 27 (Grottaferrata, Klosterbibliothek, 2 Γ VI [series IX cod. 46])

Ιερουσαλήμ, Πατριαρχείο, Πατριαρχική Βιβλιοθήκη
Ιερά Μονή Αγίου Σάββα
See Jerusalemn, Bibl. Mar-Saba
432: 29
481: 29
Πανάγιος Τάφος
See Jerusalem, Bibl. patriarch.
102: 29
148: 29
Πατριαρχείο
68: 28 (Jerusalem, Bibl. d. Hl. Kreuzes 68)
Ιερά Μονή Τιμίου Σταυρού
85: 29 (Jerusalem, Bibl. d. Hl. Kreuzes 85)

Jena, Thüringer Universitäts- und Landesbibliothek
See Jena, Universitätsbibliothek
Aldina c. nott. Cornarii: 28
Ms. G.B. f. 31: 49 ([Moskau, Synodialbibl., ?])

Καλλονή Λέσβου, Βιβλιοθήκη τῆς τοῦ Λειμῶνος Μονῆς
See Lesbos, Βιβλ. τῆς τοῦ Λειμῶνος Μονῆς
175: 32

København, Det Kongelige Bibliotek
See Kopenhagen, Königl. Bibliothek, and Bibl. Univ.
e don. var.
14, 2°: 30 (Bibl. Univ., e donatione variorum Fol. 14)
29, 2°: 59 (Padua. Bibl. Joann. Rhodiis)
42, 4°: 30 (Bibl. Univ., e donatione variorum 4° 42), 59 (Padua, Bibl. Joann. Rhodii)
GkS
224, 2°: 30 (Königl. Bibliothek, Hauniens. ant. fund. reg. 224)
225, 2°: 30 (Königl. Bibliothek, Hauniens. ant. fund. reg. 225)
1648, 4°: 30 (Königl. Bibliothek, Hauniens. ant. fund. reg. 1648)

London, British Library
See London, British Museum
- Additional
  - See Addit. or Adit. (Brit. Mus.)
  - 6898: 36 (Addit. 6898), 102 (Venedig, Monast. S. Michaelis prope Murianum 93)
  - 10,058: 36
  - 11,888: 36
  - 17,900: 36
  - 28,830: 37
- *Arundeliani*
  - 537: 37 (Arundel. –)
- *Burneiani*
  - 94: 37
  - 523: 37
- *Harleiani*
  - 5611: 37
  - 5625: 37
  - 5626: 37
  - 5651: 37
  - 5652: 38
  - 6305: 38
- Royal
  - 16.C.xi: 38

London, Wellcome Library
- MS. MSL
- See London, Medical Society
- 52 A&B: 39 (HH i 21. 22 = We 28. 29)
- 60: 38 (HHi 17 = We 30)
- 83: 38 (–)

Madrid, Biblioteca nacional
See Madrid, Nationalbibliothek
- 4631: 39 (4631 [N 110])
- 4783: 39 (4783 [olim O 67])

Messina, Biblioteca Regioniale Univesitaria Giacomo Longo di Messina
- S. Salvatore
  - 84: 45 (Messina, Universität 84)
  - F 4/4B: 45 (Messina, Universität 111)

Modena, Biblioteca Estense Universitaria
See Modena, Bibl. Estense
α.G.3.11: 46 (211 [III G 7])
α.G.3.12: 47 (213), (213 [III G 9])
α.J.6.28: 48 (240 [III F 17])
α.O.4.6: 47 (218 [II H 3])
α.O.4.7: 47 (217 [II H 2])
α.O.4.9: 47 (216 [II H 1])
α.O.4.11: 48 (219 [II H 4])
α.O.4.12: 48 (226 [II H 11])
α.P.5.17: 46 (115 [II D 16])
α.P.5.18: 46 (107 [II D 8])
α.P.5.20: 46 (109 [II D 10])
α.U.9.4: 45 (61 [III B 9])
α.U.9.23: 46 (97 [III C 18])
α.V.6.12: 46 (210 [III G 6])
α.V.7.4: 46 (175 [II F 10])
α.V.7.18: 46 (151 [II E 18])
α.W.2.9: 45 (78 [II C 11])
α.W.3.12: 48 (237 [III G 18])

Москва (Moskva), Государственный Исторический Музей (ГИМ), Синодальная Библиотека Московского Патриархата (Gosudarstvennyi Istoricheskii Muzei (GIM), Sinodalnaja Biblioteka Moskovskoi Patriarchii [State Historical Museum [GIM], Synodal Library of Moscow Patriarchate])
Синод. (Sinod.)
See Moskau, Synodialbibl.
51: 49 (Mosquenses complures), (51), (52 [*so !*]), 50 (464)
282: 50 (465)
283: 49 (Mosquenses complures), (283 [= 466]), 50 (466)
292: 49 (260), 50 (292)
303: 50 (395)
507: 49 (Mosquenses complures), 51 (467)
508: 51 (468)

Москва (Moskva), Российский Государственный Архив Древних Актов (РГАДА) (Rossiiskii Gosudarsdarstvennyj Arkhiv Drevnikh Aktov [RGADA], Russian State Archive of Ancient Documents [RGADA])
Фонда 1607: Дрезденские рукописные книги (Коллекция греческих рукописей) (Fonda 1607 : Drezdenskie rukopisnye knigi [Kollektsiya grecheskikh

2159: 67
2160: 68 (2160), 70 ([2169 (?)])
2161: 68
2162: 68 (2162), 75 ([2262 (?)])
2163: 68
2164: 68 (2164), 70 ([2167 (?)]),([2169 (?)]), 82 (2664)
2165: 69
2166: 67 ([2156 (?)]), 69 (2166)
2167: 65 ([2137 (?)]), 67 ([2157 (?)]), 69 (2167)
2168: 70
2169: 70
2170: 70 (2170), ([2170 (?)])
2171: 71
2172: 71
2173: 64 ([2123 (?)]), 71 (2173)
2174: 71
2175: 71
2176: 71
2177: 71
2178: 71
2183: 72
2195: 72
2207: 72
2210: 72
2219: 72
2224: 72
2228: 72
2229: 72
2230: 73 (2230), ([2230])
2232: 73
2237: 73
2238: 72 ([2208 (?)]), 73 (2238)
2240: 73
2246: 73
2247: 73 ([2245 (?)]), 74 (2247), ([2247 (?)])
2248: 73 ([2245 (?)]), 74 (2248), (2248 [?])
2253: 74
2255: 74
2256: 74
2257: 74
2260: 68 (2160 (?)]), 75 (2260), 78 ([2280 (?)])

Catalogue of Manuscripts

Notes for consultation

The catalogue that follows collects and exactly reproduces all the data presented for the Greek manuscripts with Galenic content listed in Diels. Each manuscript received an entry in which data are divided in two major parts: identification (followed by possible annotations) and contents[1].

Identifications of the manuscripts comprise a city and library name, a collection when appropriate, and a shelfmark. City names are mostly in German, whereas library names are either in German or in the original language (and in the Greek alphabet for several, but not all, of the libraries in Greece). The library names used by Diels do not always follow the actual form they had in Diels' time and, whatever their exactness, they are often in an abbreviated form. Collection names are either those of the libraries (often in an abbreviated form) or Latin adjectives formed on the name of the city. Shelfmarks are those used when Diels was compiled or sometimes, earlier ones, or even both. For some manuscripts, erroneous shelfmarks provided in the first two issues of Diels are corrected in the *Nachtrag* (Supplement). In some cases, Diels does not provide a shelfmark, but only a reference to a citation in an earlier catalogue or a more recent publication. For several items, all or some of these data (specifically the shelfmarks) appear between brackets in Diels (sometimes also with a question mark within the brackets) to indicate that they are reproduced from Ackermann (1791 and 1796) or Littré (1839–1861)[2]. The year or, in most cases, the century of copy of the manuscripts follows. For several manuscripts this chronological indication varies from one occurrence to another. All such divergent estimates are provided here in chronological order. In the catalogue contained in this volume, all these data form the first line of the entry devoted to each manuscript; they are printed in boldface for the purposes of easy and direct consultation. Notes about the possible untraceability and the state of preservation of some manuscripts, as well as possible corrections of shelfmark and time of copy provided in the *Nachtrag* (Supplement) are reproduced in the next line, printed in italic.

When necessary, the identification of the manuscripts is followed (on the next line) by annotations providing the correspondence between Diels' and current identi-

1 Only manuscripts that have been preserved and precisely identified are listed here. Items lost (already in Diels' time or later), destroyed (including because of the two World Wars), missing, or mentioned in Diels, but not precisely identified as per the *Census*, have been omitted. They appear, however, in the catalogue of manuscripts in tome 5.

2 See p. 2 in the 1905 issue for an explanation of the brackets.

fication of the manuscripts since several Diels identifiers do not correspond to their actual or current equivalent (from the city names in German to possible changes of shelfmarks). Correspondences (particularly of shelfmarks) that could not be established with a degree of certainty are introduced by a question mark. All correspondences reproduce those provided in the *Census of Greek Medical Manuscripts* (2016), which is referenced between parentheses after the current identification. To avoid repetition among the entries when several manuscripts appear in the same library or collection, Diels' and current names are provided only once, at the beginning of the section of the catalogue devoted to the library or the collection.

A special case is that of the manuscripts listed in Diels under different shelfmarks or with a shelfmark between brackets. Each distinct shelfmark in Diels has received an entry. However, all such entries include a reference to the manuscripts they refer to and, conversely, they are referred to in the entry of the manuscripts they are related to. These cross-references follow the identification of the manuscripts (Diel's and current). Shelfmarks (or other identifiers) referred to are printed in boldface to allow for easy cross-referencing.

The second and most substantial part of each entry details the contents of the manuscripts. All the texts included in Diels (and only those) are listed here as in the manuscripts, with the following descriptors[3]: the folios where they appear or their sequential number in the manuscripts (in both cases between parentheses), the title of the work (in italic), and any possible notes of commentary between parentheses (*incipit*, lacunae, *desinit*, source, comparison with other texts, or any other philological or textual peculiarity as identified in Diels, sometimes with the name of Diels' collaborator who provided the information). References to other manuscripts (sometimes without precise shelfmark in Diels) have been made explicit (via shelfmark between brackets) to allow for cross-referencing. The asterisk that follows the title of some works in Diels to indicate a fragmentary text has been replaced by the explicit mention *Frgm.* References to the parts and pages of Diels' catalogue, and mentions of collations made or owned by Diels' collaborators have been omitted, as have also been some notes historico-critical in nature.

3 Galen's name has been systematically omitted.

Amsterdam

[Amsterdam, Universitäts-Bibliothek, Amstelodam. ?].
= Oxford, Bodleian Library, MS. D'Orville 3 (*Census*: 9, nr [0001]). See below p. 59.

Linguarum sive dictionum exoletarum Hippocratis explicatio.

Athen, Nationalbibl.
Αθνήνα, Εθνική Βιβλιοθήκη της Ελλάδος ΕΒΕ

Athen, Nationalbibl., 1479; s. XIX.

Dioscurides, Galenos, Paulus Aegineta, *Excerpta/Iatrosophia* (Ἰατροσόφιον ἀπηθισμένον ἀπὸ Γαλ., Παύλου τοῦ Αἰγ. ... καὶ Δ.).

Athen, Nationalbibl., 1491; s. XVIII.

(nr 1) *De differentiis morborum.*
(nr 2) *De morborum causis.*
(nr 3) *De symptomatum differentiis.*
(nr 4. 5) *De symptomatum causis libri III.*

Athen, Nationalbibl., 1493; s. XII ex.

(nr 1) *De remediis parabilibus libri III* (Frgm. ex libris I et II).
(nr 3–5) *De animalibus noxiis* (nr 3: Θεραπεία πρὸς τὰς ἀπὸ τῶν ἰοβόλων ἑρπετῶν ἱπταμένων καὶ ἐνύδρων θηρίων πληγάς; nr 4: Περὶ ζῴων φθαρτικῶν καὶ αἵματος, σπερμάτων τε καὶ ῥιζῶν καὶ μεταλλικῶν καὶ λοιπῶν θανατηφόρων καὶ τῆς τούτων θεραπείας; nr 5: Περὶ ζῴων φθαρτικῶν).

Athen, Nationalbibl., 1494; s. XVIII.

(nr 1) *De methodo medendi libri XIV* (Frgm. Εἰσαγωγὴ ἐκ τῆς μεγάλης θεραπευτικῆς).

Athen, Nationalbibl., 1502; s. XVIII.

(nr 1) *Introductio sive medicus.*

Athos, Βιβλ. Μον. Διονυσίου
Now Άγιον Όρος, Ιερά Μονή Διονυσίου

Athos, Βιβλ. Μον. Διονυσίου, 3701. 167; s. XV.
Now 59 (*Census*: 16, nr [0028]).

De hominis natura testamentum. De victu singulis mensibus servando I (Inc. Ἐγὼ Γαληνὸς πεπειραμένος πάνυ τοῦ τῶν ἀνθρώπων ἤθους).

Athos, Βιβλ. Μον. Ἰβήρων
Now Άγιον Όρος, Ιερά Μονή Ιβήρων

Athos, Βιβλ. Μον. Ἰβήρων, 4271. 151; s. XV.
= 151 (4271).

(f. 19) *De remediis parabilibus libri III* (Libri II inscr. Γαλ. θεραπευτικὴ διαφόρων νόσων διὰ τῶν εὐπορίστων φαρμάκων. Inc. Περὶ τῆς ἐξεκκαύσεως κεφαλαλγίας. Expl. γάλα ἵστησιν).
(f. 71 A. 74 A. 80 A) *De animalibus noxiis* (= Athen. [1493] no. 3–5; f. 71 A Inc. Σφηκῶν καὶ μελισσῶν ἁρμόζει. f. 74 Inc. Ζῷα μὲν οὖν ἐστι φθαρτικά. f. 80 Inc. Περὶ βοτανῶν. Βοτάνη ἀγριοπήγανον. Αὕτη ποιεῖ πρὸς τὰς ἐμπνευματώσεις).
(f. 128 a) *Ad Glauconem de medendi methodo libri II.*
(f. 176 A) *Remedia* (Ζουλαπίου σύνθεσις. Inc. Ζουλάπιον εἰς βῆχα).
(f. 224) *Lexicon botanicum* (Inc. Ἄρκευστον ἢ καντζάρου ἢ κέδρος. Expl. Σισύμβριον τὸ βάρσαμον).

Athos, Βιβλ. Μον. Ἰβήρων, 4284. 164; s. XIII.
= 164 (4284) (*Census*: 19, nr [0045]).

De methodo medendi libri XIV.
Ars medica (Frgm. »Τάξις τῶν πραγματειῶν τοῦ Γ. κατὰ αὐτὸν ἐν τῷ τέλει τοῦ Μικρὰ τέχνη ἐπιγεγραμμένου βιβλίου«).

Athos, Βιβλ. Μον. Ἰβήρων, 4294. 174; s. XVII.
= 174 (4294) (*Census*: 19, nr [0046]).

(f. 46b [463 ?]) **Hippokrates/Galenos**, *Jatrosophium* (Ἰατροσόφιον ἐκλελεγμ. ὑπὸ πολλ. ἰατρικῶν βιβλίων Γαλ. Ἱππ. καὶ ἄλλων πολλ. σοφῶν ἰατρῶν).

Athos, Βιβλ. Μον. Ἰβήρων, 4300. 180; s. XVII.
= 180 (4300) (*Census*: 19, nr [0047]).

(f. 172) *Introductio sive medicus.*

Athos, Βιβλ. Μον. Ἰβήρων, 4304. 184; s. XIV/XV.
= 184 (4304) (*Census*: 19, nr [0051]).

(f. 130 A) *In Hippocratis librum de acutorum victu commentarii IV.*

Athos, Βιβλ. Μον. Ἰβήρων, 4309. 189; s. XIII.
= 189 (4309) (*Census*: 19, nr [0052]).

(f. 42 A) *In Hippocratis librum de acutorum victu commentarii IV.*
(f. 174 b) *De crisibus libri III.*
(f. 247 b) *De diebus decretoriis libri III.*
(f. 371 A) *De curandi ratione per venae sectionem.*

Athos, Βιβλ. Μον. Ἰβήρων, 4310. 190; s. XIII.
= 190 (4310) (*Census*: 20, nr [0053]).

(f. 115 a) *Excerpta varia.*

Athos, Βιβλ. Μον. Ἰβήρων, 4339. 219; s. XVIII.
= 219 (4339) (*Census*: 20, nr [0059]).

De antidotis libri II.
Remedia (Περὶ ἐλαίων).

Athos, Βιβλ. Μον. Ἰβήρων, 4508. 388; s. XVI.
= 388 (4508) (*Census*: 21, nr [0067]).

Remedia (Κοκκία καθαρτικὰ στομάχου καὶ κεφαλῆς).

Athos, Βιβλ. Μον. Ἰβήρων, 4655. 535; s. XVI.
= 535 (4655) (*Census*: 21, nr [0068]).

Galenos, Hippokrates, Meletius monachus, *Iatrosophia/excerpta varia* (Ἰατροσόφη ἐκλελεγμένον ὑπὸ ... Γαλ. Ἱππ. καὶ Μελ. καὶ ἄλλων δοκίμων ἰατρῶν. Cap. 1. Ὅτι ὁ κόσμος ὑπὸ τεσσάρων στοιχείων).

Athos, Βιβλ. Μον. Ἰβήρων, 4789. 669; s. XVIII.
= 669 (4789) (*Census*: 22, nr [0072]).

De anni temporibus (Ἑρμηνεία περὶ τῶν ὡρῶν καὶ ἔτους).

Athos, Βιβλ. Μον. Ἰβήρων, 5034. 914; s. XVII.
= 914 (5034) (*Census*: 22, nr [0077]).

De hominis natura testamentum. De victu singulis mensibus servando (Inc. *wie im* Athous μον. Διονυσίου [3701. 167] [above p. 6]. Expl. πρὸς ὑγείαν τοῦ σώματος τοῖς καλῶς χρωμένοις).

Athos, Βιβλ. Μον. Ἰβήρων, 5437. 1317; s. XVIII.
= 1317 (5437) (*Census*: 22, nr [0078]).

De anni temporibus (Ἰατροσόφιον Γαλ. ἰατροῦ Ἑρμηνεία. Inc. Τὸ ἔαρ ἄρχεται ἀπὸ τῆς κε΄ τοῦ μηνός).

Athos, Βιβλ. Μον. Κουτλουμουσίου
Now Άγιον Όρος, Ιερά Μονή Κουτλουμουσίου

Athos, Βιβλ. Μον. Κουτλουμουσίου, 3321. 248; s. XVII.
= 248 (3321) (*Census*: 23, nr [0080]).

Definitiones medicae (Ὅροι τῶν νοσημάτων); **Oribasius**, *Excerpta varia*.

Athos, Βιβλ. Μον. Παντελεήμονος
Now Άγιον Όρος, Ιερά Μονή Παντελεήμονος

Athos, Βιβλ. Μον. Παντελεήμονος, 5578. 72; s. XV.
= 72 (5578) (*Census*: 25, nr [0090]).

(f. 458 a) *Excerpta varia* (Γαλ. γνώμη. Inc. Ὁ γὰρ οὐκ ἐβούλετο, τοῦτο οὐκ ᾤετο).

Athos, Βιβλ. Μον. Παντελεήμονος, 5769. 262; s. XVIII.
= 262 (5769) (*Census*: 25, nr [0093]).

(f. 15 [15 A]) **Meletius monachus, Hippokrates, Galenos, Paulus Aegineta**, *Excerpta varia* (Ἰατροσόφιον ἐκλελεγμένον ὑπὸ πολλῶν ἰατρικῶν βιβλ. Γαλ. Ἱππ. Μελ. καὶ Παύλ. τοῦ Αἰγ. συγγραφὲν δὲ παρὰ Κοσμᾶ ἱερομονάχου τοῦ Μακεδόνος).

Athos, Παντοκράτορος
Now Άγιον Όρος, Ιερά Μονή Παντοκράτορος

Athos, Παντοκράτορος, 1268. 234; s. XIII.
Άγιον Όρος, Ιερά Μονή Παντοκράτορος, 234 (1268) (*Census*: 26, nr [0100]).

Excerpta varia (Inc. …κάστου ἐξα' γ' κιναμώμου. Expl. εὑρίσκονται καὶ θερμά).

Athos, Βιβλ. Μον. Ξηροποτάμου
Now Άγιον Όρος, Ιερά Μονή Ξηροποτάμου

Athos, Βιβλ. Μον. Ξηροποτάμου, 2342. 99; s. XVII.
Same as **2432. 99** below (*Census*: 26, nr [0098]).
= 99.2432.

De dolore capitis (Περὶ πόνου κεφαλῆς).

Athos, Βιβλ. Μον. Ξηροποτάμου, 2432. 99; s. XVII.
= 99 (2432) (*Census*: 26, nr [0099]).
See also **2342. 99** above.

De hominis natura testamentum. De victu singulis mensibus servando (Διαθ. … Γαλ. Ἱππ. καὶ Μελετίου π. κατασκ. ἀνθρ. κτλ.).

Berlin, Königl. Bibl.
Now Staatsbibliothek zu Berlin – Preussischer Kulturbesitz SBB-PKB

Berlin, Königl. Bibl., qu. 5 (304); s. XV/XVI.
Now Kraków, Biblioteka Jagiellońska, quarto 5 (*Census*: 33, nr [0152], 103).

(f. 53^{v}) *De hominis natura testamentum. De victu singulis mensibus servando* (*Wie im* Athous Ξηροποταμοῦ [2432. 99]) (above).

Berlin, Königl. Bibl., Hamilton. 270 (401); s. XIII.
= Ms. Ham. 270 (*Census*: 28, nr [0116]).
See also **Venedig, Bibl. monaster. S. Michaelis Venet. prope Murianum, 132** below (p. 102).

De placitis Hippocratis et Platonis libri IX (*Collation bei Petersen diss. Gotting. 1888; vgl. E. Wellmann Rhein. Mus. 40, 30 ff., Kalbfleisch diss. Berol. 1892*).

Berlin, Königl. Bibl., Phillipps.
Now Berlin, Staatsbibliothek zu Berlin – Preussischer Kulturbesitz SBB-PKB, Ms. Phill.

Berlin, Königl. Bibl., Phillipps. 1462; s. XV/XVI.
= Ms. Phill. 1462 (*Census*: 29, nr [0118]).

(f. 410) *De hominis natura testamentum. De victu singulis mensibus servando I* (Inc. *und* Expl. *wie im* Athous μον. Ἰβήρων [5034. 914] [above p. 8]).

Berlin, Königl. Bibl., Phillipps. 1524 (ol. Meerm. 214); s. XV, XVI.
= Ms. Phill. 1524 (*Census*: 29, nr [0120]).

(f. 41) *De pulsibus ad tirones* (Expl. σκεψώμεθα = K. VIII 484, 9).

Berlin, Königl. Bibl., Phillipps. 1525 (ol. Meerm. 215); s. XVI.
= Ms. Phill. 1525 (*Census*: 29, nr [0121]).

Linguarum sive dictionum exoletarum Hippocratis explicatio (Expl. mutil. ψαφερον ψαδυρὸν ψέφαρα).

Berlin, Königl. Bibl., Phillipps. 1526 (ol. Meerm. 216); s. XVI.
= Ms. Phill. 1526 (*Census*: 29, nr [0122]).

Introductio sive medicus (Non sine lacunis).
Definitiones medicae (Sine titulo).

Berlin, Königl. Bibl., Phillipps. 1527 (ol. Meerm. 217); s. XVI.
= Ms. Phill. 1527 (*Census*: 29, nr [0123]).

(f. 1^v–2^r) *De usu partium corporis humani libri XVII.*

Berlin, Königl. Bibl., Phillipps. 1529 (ol. Meerm. 220); s. XVI.
= Ms. Phill. 1529 (*Census*: 30, nr [0125]).

(f. 1) *De compositione medicamentorum per genera libri VII* (Inc. μὴ δ' ὅλως δάκνοντα = K. XIII 499, 10 [lib. II 5]. Expl. = lib. VII 16, K. XIII 1047).

Berlin, Königl. Bibl., Phillipps. 1566 (ol. Meerm. 269); s. XVI.
= Ms. Phill. 1566 (*Census*: 31, nr [0141]).

De sanitate tuenda libri VI (Frgm. = K. VI 281 sq.).
(f. 6) *De hominis natura testamentum. De victu singulis mensibus servando.*
(f. 14) *De compositione medicamentorum secundum locos libri X* (Lib. X cap. 2.).
(f. 19) *De pulsibus ad Antonium* (in fine pauca omissa).

Berlin, Königl. Bibl., Phillipps. 1567 (ol. Meerm. 270); s. XVI.
= Ms. Phill. 1567 (*Census*: 31, nr [0142]).

(f. 1) *De ossibus ad tirones.*

Berlin, Königl. Bibl., Phillipps. 1570; s. XVI.
= Ms. Phill. 1570 (*Census*: 31, nr [0144]).

(f. 63) *Lexicon botanicum* (Inc. Ἀκταία · ἡ κουφοξυλαία. Expl. ὤκιμον τὸ βασιλικόν).

Berlin, Königl. Bibl., Phillipps. 1571; s. XVI.
= Ms. Phill. 1571 (*Census*: 32, nr [0145]).

(f. 3) *De venae sectione* (K. XIX 519–528) (Initium opusc. = K. XIX 519–521, 15).

Berlin, Königl. Bibl., Phillipps. 1577 (Meerm. 287); s. XV.
= Ms. Phill. 1577 (*Census*: 32, nr [0147]).

(f. 87) *Prognostica de decubitu ex mathematica scientia* (Inc. Συσχηματίζεται = K. XIX 532, 10–533, 6 γνωρίζεται).

Berlin, Königl. Bibl., Phillipps. 1991 (ol. Meerm. 218); s. XVI.
= Ms. Phill. 1991 (*Census*: 33, nr [0151]).

(f. 2) *De differentiis morborum* (Inc. Τὸ δὲ στέγνωσις = K. VI 842, 2).
(f. 13^{v}) *De morborum causis* (Inscr. Συμπτωμάτων [superscriptum: νοσημάτων] διαφορᾶς λόγος β').
(f. 27^{v}) *De symptomatum differentiis.*
(f. 41^{v}) *De symptomatum causis libri III.*

Bern, Stadtbibliothek
Now Burgerbibliothek Bern/Bibliothèque de la Bourgeoisie de Berne

Bern, Stadtbibliothek, 691; s. XV–XVI.

(f. 80–81) *De propriorum animi cuiuslibet affectuum dignotione et curatione* (Frgm. Inc. Οὐ φαίνεσθαι χρὴ τοῖς τοιούτοις. Expl. ἀπὸ στόματος ὕστερον).

Bologna, Bibl. Universitaria

Bologna, Bibl. Universitaria, Bonon. 1808; s. XV.

(f. 64) *De ponderibus et mensuris* (Inc. Ὁ σταθμὸς βάρει. Expl. τὴν ῥοπὴν διαφορᾶ).
(f. 116) *De carbunculis.*
(f. 118) *De erysipelate.*
(f. 123^{v}) *Remedia* (Ἡ διὰ πτέργης [sic !] · μάλαγμα πηγανηρόν).
(f. 143) *De stomacho* (Περὶ ἀτονίας στομάχου καὶ ὑπτιασμοῦ καὶ ἀνατροπῆς).
(f. 213) *De contusionibus.*
(f. 270^{v}) *De nimia seminis profusione.*
(f. 293^{v}) *De lepra alba.*
(f. 299^{v}) *Remedia* (Ξηρὰ ἀνακαθαρτικὰ καὶ σαρκωτικὰ κεφαλικὰ λεγόμενα).
(f. 301^{v}) *De vulneribus* (Π. ἑλκῶν τῶν μὴ κακοήθων οὐλῆς δεομένων).

Bologna, Bibl. Universitaria, Bonon. 2678 (ol. 228); s. XV.

(f. 67) *De simplicium medicamentorum temperamentis et facultatibus libri XI* (Libri VI–XI).

Bologna, Bibl. Universitaria, Bonon. 3632; s. XV.

(f. 63^{v}) *De pulsibus ad tirones* (Frgm.).
(f. 63^{v}) *De pulsibus ad Antonium* (Frgm.).
(f. 129–131) *Definitiones medicae.*
(f. 132) *De febribus* (De febrium differentiis).
(f. 132) *De differentiis febrium libri II* (Frgm. Exc. de febrium differentiis [?]).
(f. 205) *Remedia* (Περὶ τῶν ἱερῶν καὶ πικρῶν ἀντιδότων cap. ιθ').
(f. 260) *De succedaneis liber.*
(f. 261) *De ponderibus et mensuris* (Frgm.).
(f. 265) *De lacte.*

Bologna, Bibl. Universitaria, Bonon. 3636; s. XIV–XV.

(f. 1) *Ars medica.*
(f. 120) *De optima ventris concoctione.*
(f. 125–126) *De urinis* (Inc. Ἄριστον οὖρόν ἐστι. Expl. τότε καὶ συνίσταται τὸ οὖρον).
(f. 126) *De humoribus* (Σημεῖα κράσεως χυμῶν. Inc. Σκεπτέον ἐπὶ πάντων. Expl. κατὰ φύσιν οὐδέν τι τούτων ποιήσει).
(f. 126) *De temperamentis* (Frgm. σημεῖα κράσεως χυμῶν. Inc. Σκεπτέον ἐστὶ πάντων. Expl. κατὰ φύσιν οὐδένα τούτων ποιήσει).
(f. 129ᵛ) *De curandi ratione per venae sectionem* (cap. IV–XXI. Inc. Ὅτι τοῖς τὰ συνήθη πράττουσι. Expl. ἀλλὰ τηρεῖν καὶ αὖθις ἐπαφαιρεῖν).
(f. 133) *De curandi ratione per venae sectionem* (cap. XXII).

Bologna, Bibl. Universitaria, Bonon. 3637; s. XIV.

(f. 2) *De foetuum formatione* (Περὶ τῆς τοῦ ἀνθρώπου διαπλάσεως).

Brüssel, Königl. Bibl.
Now Bruxelles, Bibliothèque royale de Belgique

Brüssel, Königl. Bibl., Bruxell. 11345–48; s. XVI.

(f. 25) *Linguarum sive dictionum exoletarum Hippocratis explicatio.*

Cairo

Cairo, Patriarch. Alexandrin., 46 (*bei* Coxe, Mss. gr. of the Levant); s. XV.
= Αλεξάνδρεια (الإسكندرية), Πατριαρχείο, Πατριαρχική Βιβλιοθήκη Αλεξανδρείας, 36 (?) (*Census*: 39, nr [0181]).

Excerpta varia (Περὶ ὑποκρισέων [sic]).

Cambridge, Caius Coll.
Now Cambridge, Gonville and Caius College

Cambridge, Caius Coll., 47; s. XV.
Now 47/24 (*Census*: 40, nr [0183]).
See also **[946]** below and possibly **[6605]** (p. 15).

(f. 0) *De usu partium corporis humani libri XVII* (Libri VI [init. mut.]–XI).
(f. 1) *Methodi medendi libri XIV* (Lib. I–VI in fine mutil.).
(nr III) *De placitis Hippocratis et Platonis libri IX.*
(nr IV) *De XII portis* (Frgm. Inc. in porta XVII καὶ βλάβης εἶδον. Expl. in porta XIX ἰατροὶ τοῦ κόπτειν τὴν αἶεραν).

Cambridge, Caius Coll., 76; s. XV/XVI.
Now 76/43 (*Census*: 40, nr [0185]).
See also **[949]** below (p. 15).

(f. 142 und f. 143) *De differentiis febrium libri II* (Frgm. l. I ex. Inc. προεξηρασμένον τὸ τῆς καρδίας σῶμα. Expl. πυρετῶν ἁπάσας ἐροῦμεν διαφοράς).

Cambridge, Caius Coll., 355; s. XV/XVI.
Now 355/582 (*Census*: 40, nr [0187]).
See also **[948]** below (p. 15).

(f. 1) *De symptomatum differentiis.*
(f. 17) *De symptomatum causis libri III.*
(f. 135) *De usu pulsuum.*
(f. 151) *Definitiones medicae* (Γαλ. περὶ ὅρων ἰατρικῶν. Inc. Ὅρα σοφὴν σύνταξιν ἐ⟨ν⟩τέρων ὅλων. Expl. τοῖς σώμασιν ἐκ τῶν λαμβανομένων τροφῶν).

Cambridge, Caius Coll., 360; s. XVI.
Now 360/587 (*Census*: 40, nr [0188]).

(f. 1) *De elementis secundum Hippocratem.*
(p. 85) *De facultatibus naturalibus.*
(p. 161) *Methodi medendi libri XIV* (Lib. VI–XIV).

[Cambridge, Caius Coll., 946; s. –].
= part of **47** above (*Census*: 40–41, nr [0189]).
Now 47/24.

De usu partium corporis humani libri XVII (imperf.).
De abortivo foetu.

[Cambridge, Caius Coll., 948; s. –].
= part of **355** above (p. 14) (*Census*: 42, nr [0190]).
Now 355/582.

Definitiones medicae.

[Cambridge, Caius Coll., 949; s. –].
= part of **76** above (p. 14) (*Census*: 42, nr [0191]).
Now 76/43.

De differentiis febrium libri II.

[Cambridge, Caius Coll., 6605; s. –].
Possibly same as **47** and **[946]** above (p. 14) (*Census*: 43–44, nr [0196]).

De abortivo foetu.

Cambridge, Cantabrig. Bibl. Univ.
Now Cambridge, University Library

Cambridge, Cantabrig. Bibl. Univ., F. F. 3. 30; s. XVI.
Now Cambridge University Library Ff. 3. 30.

(nr 2) *De simplicium medicamentorum temperamentis et facultatibus libri XI* (Frgm. Ἀπὸ τῶν τοῦ Γαλ. ἁπλῶν ἐκλογή τινων κεφαλαίων κτέ.).
(nr 5) *De diaeta et morbis curandis.*

Carpentras

Carpentras, Bibl. Inguimbertine, nr. 1774 (P., V/ P. V.); s. XVII.

(f. 313) *De ponderibus et mensuris.*

Cheltenham

Cheltenham, Phillipps., 4614; s. XV (XIV), XV (XIV ?).
Now New Haven, Yale University, Beinecke Rare Book and Manuscript Library, MS 1121 (*Census*: 51, nr [0215]).

(nr 5) *De optima corporis nostri constitutione.*

(f. 1) *De temperamentis* (Inc. = K. I 635, 9).
(f. 15ᵛ) *De facultatibus naturalibus.*
(f. 54ᵛ) *De inaequali intemperie.*
(f. 60) *De bono habitu.*
(f. 62) *De difficultate respirationis libri III.*
(f. 107) *Ad Glauconem de medendi methodo libri II.*
(f. 141) *De alimentorum facultatibus libri III.*

Cheltenham, Phillipps., 6665–6765; s. XII.
Now Munich, Bayerische Staatsbibliothek, *Monacensis graecus* 633 (*Census*: 51, nr [0216], 157).
Same as **6774** below.

(nr 2) *De simplicium medicamentorum temperamentis et facultatibus libri XI* (Frgm. *Wie im* Cantabrig. [Bibl. Univ. F. F. 3. 30] [above p. 15]. Inc. Ἀβρότονον · θερμόν ἐστι καὶ ξηρόν. Expl. πεπονθόσι τὴν κύστιν καὶ τοῖς λιθιῶσιν).

Cheltenham, Phillipps., 6774 (ol. Meerm. 298); s. XII.
Same as **6665–6765** above.
Now Munich, Bayerische Staatsbibliothek, *Monacensis graecus* 633 (*Census*: 51–52, nr [0218]).

De simplicium medicamentorum temperamentis et facultatibus libri XI (Frgm. *Wie im* Cantabr. [Bibl. Univ. F. F. 3. 30]) (above p. 15).

Cheltenham, Phillipps., 23007; s. XV.
Now divided in three manuscripts (see *Census*: 52, nr [0220])).

Paris, Chicago, and New York, Les Enluminures, TM 540.
Provo, Brigham Young University, Lee Library, L. Tom Perry Special Collections,vault 091 G13 1475.
Paris, private collection.

De historia philosopha.

Cheltenham, Phillipps., 24, 386; s. XV.
Now Bethesda, National Library of Medicine, MS. 82 *Census* (*Census*: 52, nr [0221]).

(f. 1) *Synopsis librorum suorum sedecim de pulsibus.*

Dresden, Königl. Bibl.
Now Sächsische Landesbibliothek – Staats- und Universitätsbibliothek Dresden

Dresden, Königl. Bibl., Da 1; s. XV.
Now Москва (Moskva), Российский Государственный Архив Древних Актов (РГАДА) (Rossiiskii Gosudarstvennyi Arkhiv Drevnikh Aktov [RGADA], Russian State Archive of Ancient Documents [RGADA]), Фонд (Fond.) 1607, Dresden Da 01 (*Census*: 57–58, nr [0223]).

(f. 1) *Introductio sive medicus.*
(f. 24ᵛ) *Ars medica.*

Dresden, Königl. Bibl., Aldina.

Galen, *Opera varia* (»Galeni operum exemplar Aldinum ... hac re conspicuum, quod et in textu ipso nonnulla atramento sunt correcta et in margine librorum plurimorum adnotantur argumenta brevia, versiones latinae, variae denique lectiones haud paucae«. *Der III. Band fehlt. Vgl.* Ilberg, Philol. 48. N. F. II S. 57–66).

Escurial
Now San Lorenzo de El Escorial, Biblioteca del Real Monastero de San Lorenzo del Escorial

Escurial, Scorial. III. R. 3; s. XI.
= R.III.3 (*Census*: 62, nr [0238]).

(f. 138) *De atra bile* (Frgm. Ἀντίδοτον Γαλ. ... ὠφελοῦν εἰς τὴν μέλαιναν χολὴν καὶ εἰς τὴν ξανθήν. Expl. ἔχεις καὶ θέλης. ἐστὶν γὰρ ὠφελιμώτατον).
(f. 138) *Remedia* (Ἀντίδοτον Γαλ. ... ὠφελοῦν εἰς τὴν μέλαιναν χολὴν καὶ εἰς τὴν ξανθήν. Expl. ἔχεις καὶ θέλης. ἐστὶν γὰρ ὠφελιμώτατον).

Escurial, Scorial. C. II. 11; s. XV.
Same as **Σ. II. 11** below (p. 18) (*Census*: 62, nr [0239]).

(f. 37) *De simplicium medicamentorum temperamentis et facultatibus libri XI.*

Escurial, Scorial. C. III. 17; s. XVI.
Same as **Σ. III. 17** below (*Census*: 62, nr [0240]).

(f. 36) *De simplicium medicamentorum temperamentis et facultatibus libri XI* (Libri I–V c. lacunis).

Escurial, Scorial. Σ. II. 5; s. XV.

(f. 8) *De symptomatum differentiis* (Expl. εἰρήσεται κατὰ τὸν ἑξῆς λόγον).
(f. 25) *De symptomatum causis libri III.*
(f. 73 *und* 178–183) *In Hippocratis librum de acutorum victu commentarii IV.*

Escurial, Scorial. Σ. II. 11; s. XV.
See also **C.II.11** above (p. 17).

(f. 1) *Introductio sive medicus.*
(f. 32) *In Hippocratis de humoribus librum commentarii III.*

Escurial, Scorial. Σ. III. 17; s. XVI.
See also **C.III.17** above.

(f. 25) *Introductio sive medicus* (Frgm.).
(f. 32) *De humoribus.*
(f. 94–101 [»quae ponenda sunt ante f. 25«]) *Introductio sive medicus* (Frgm.).
(f. 110) *De urinis* (Inc. Τὸ φυσικὸν οὖρον ἔνε ξανθόν. Expl. πάσχει τὰ νεῦρα σημαίνει).
(f. 114v) *Lexicon botanicum* (Inc. *wie im* Athous [Μον. Ἰβήρων 4271. 151] [above p. 6]. Expl. ἡ ῥίζα ὡς ἂν κρομιδίου).

Escurial, Scorial. T. III. 7; s. XIII.

(f. 1) *De musculorum dissectione* (Περὶ μυῶν. Inc. Τοῦ λιχανοῦ δακτύλου μετακάρπιον. Expl. περὶ μὲν οὖν τῆς τῶν μυῶν ἀνατομῆς ἱκανὰ τὰ εἰρημένα. *Vgl.* Costomiris Rev. d. étud. gr. II [1889] p. 374).
(f. 21) *De venarum arteriarumque dissectione* (Περὶ φλεβῶν. Inc. Περὶ φλεβῶν ἀνατομῆς μέλλοντες ἐξηγήσασθαι. Expl. ἐφεξῆς δὲ περὶ τῶν ἀρτηριῶν ἐροῦμεν).
(f. 28) *De venarum arteriarumque dissectione* (Περὶ ἀρτηριῶν. Inc. Ἀρχὴ μὲν τούτων ἐστὶν ἡ ἀριστερὰ κοιλία τῆς καρδίας. Expl. κατασχίζεται εἰς τὸ πᾶν σῶμα).
(f. 29v) *De nervorum dissectione* (Περὶ νεύρων. Inc. Ὅτι μὲν οὐδὲν τῶν τοῦ ζῴου μορίων. Expl. συμπράξαντος ἡμᾶς ἀριθμῆσαι ταῦτα).
(f. 34. 57v) *De motu musculorum libri II.*
(f. 73) *De ossibus ad tirones.*

(f. 90) *De musculorum dissectione* (Π. μυῶν ἀνατ. τ. εἰσαγομ.).
(f. 129) *De nervorum dissectione* (Inscr. Inc. Expl. wie gewöhnlich).
(f. 137ᵛ, 150) *De venarum arteriarumque dissectione.*

Escurial, Scorial. Υ. III. 14; s. XV.

(f. 49ᵛ) *De urinis* (Inc. Οὖρον ἄριστον μέν ἐστι πρῶτον μὲν ὁποῖον τὸ κατὰ φύσιν).
f. 238) *De succedaneis liber* (Expl. ἀντὶ χολῆς ἔχεος).

Escurial, Scorial. Υ. III. 17; s. XVI.

(f. 127) *Hippocratis aphorismi et Galeni in eos commentarii VII.*
(f. 135) *In Hippocratis prognosticum commentarii III.*

Escurial, Scorial. Φ. III. 7; s. XIV.

(f. 9) *In Hippocratis prognosticum commentarii III.*
(f. 67) *Hippocratis aphorismi et Galeni in eos commentarii VII.*

Escurial, Scorial. Φ III 11; s. XIV. XV.
Same as Φ**. III. 11** below.

(f. 16) *De usu pulsuum.*

Escurial, Scorial. Φ. III. 11; s. XIV–XV, XIV. XV, XIV *und* XV.
See also **Φ III 11** above.

(f. 40) *De urinis compendium* (fin. mutil.; *vgl.* f. 47).
(f. 43ᵛ) *De typis.*
(f. 47) *Introductio sive medicus* (Frgm. περὶ τοῦ πόσοι εἰσὶν οἱ συστησάμενοι τὴν ἐμπειρικήν = K. XIV 683).
(f. 60–66) *De simplicium medicamentorum temperamentis et facultatibus libri XI* (Frgm. Libri X. XI 1–11).
(f. 71) *De differentiis morborum* (Frgm.).
(f. 73) *De morborum causis* (Frgm. Π. αἰτίας νοσημάτων).
(f. 73ᵛ) *De symptomatum differentiis* (Frgm.).
(f. 76ᵛ *und* 78) *De symptomatum causis libri III* (Frgm. ex libr. II et III).
(f. 80) *Ad Glauconem de medendi methodo libri II* (Frgm. ex l. I).

Escurial, Scorial. Φ. III. 12; s. XV.

(f. 8ᵛ) *De urinis* (Inc. Σημεῖον ἐσχάτης ἀπεψίας. Expl. καὶ ἀσθένειαν ἐκ χρονίου νοσήματος).

Florenz, Bibl. Mediceo Laurentiana
Firenze, Biblioteca Medicea Laurenziana

Florenz, Bibl. Mediceo Laurentiana, Conventi soppressi 163; s. XVI.

(f. 5) *Galeni et Simplicii testimonia de Epicteto.*

[Florenz, Bibl. Mediceo Laurentiana, Laurent. ap. Bandini III 122].
= **plut. 74, 19** below (p. 24) (*Census*: 68, nr [0286]).

De lacte.

Florenz, Bibl. Mediceo Laurentiana, Laurent. plut. 28, 13; s. XIV.

(f. 224^{v}) *Prognostica de decubitu ex mathematica scientia* (Expl. ἀναιρεθήσονται γάρ).

Florenz, Bibl. Mediceo Laurentiana, Laurent. plut. 28, 14; s. XIV ex., XIV.

(f. 154^{v}) *Prognostica de decubitu ex mathematica scientia* (*verloren gegangen*; vgl. Catal. cod. astrol. I p. 25).

Florenz, Bibl. Mediceo Laurentiana, Laurent. plut. 28, 34; s. XI.

(f. 5) *De chirurgorum operationibus et de decubitu infirmorum* (Expl. αἴτια τῶν νόσων ἐντεῦθεν γνωρίζεται).
(f. 5 [hinter] [= f. 5^{v}]) *Prognostica de decubitu ex mathematica scientia.*

Florenz, Bibl. Mediceo Laurentiana, Laurent. plut. 56, 15; s. XV.

(p. 141) *Quod animi mores corporis temperamenta sequantur.*
(p. 206 b) *De partibus philosophiae* (Desin. imperf.).

Florenz, Bibl. Mediceo Laurentiana, Laurent. plut. 57 (?), 19; s. XIV.
= ? plut. 7.19 (*Census*: 71, nr [0300]).

(p. 224 b) *De ponderibus et mensuris.*

Florenz, Bibl. Mediceo Laurentiana, Laurent. plut. 58, 2; s. XV.

(p. 78) *De historia philosopha.*

Florenz, Bibl. Mediceo Laurentiana, Laurent. plut. 59, 14; s. XIII, XV.
Dieses Werk (= Philaretus, *De pulsibus*) *von einer Hand des XIII (!) Saec.*; f. 171v (= Galenos, *De pulsibus ad Antonium*) *andere Hand*; *sonst* s. XV.

(p. 97) *De typis.*
(p. 101) *Galeni in Hippocratis de natura hominis lib. commentarii II.*
(p. 151) *In Hippocratis vel Polybi opus de salubri victus ratione privatorum commentarius.*
(f. 171v) *De pulsibus ad Antonium* (Inscr. Ποίημα μικρὸν φιλαρέτου περὶ σφυγμῶν πρὸς Ἀντώνιον φιλομαθῆ καὶ φίλον αὐτοῦ. *Also hier unter Philarets Namen !*).
(f. 178) *Synopsis librorum suorum sedecim de pulsibus.*
(p. 213) *De foetuum formatione.*

[Florenz, Bibl. Mediceo Laurentiana, Laurent. plut. 74, (?)].
= (?) **plut. 74, 5** below (p. 22) (*Census*: 74, nr [0312]).

De morborum temporibus.

Florenz, Bibl. Mediceo Laurentiana, Laurent. plut. 74, 1; s. XV.

(f. 1v) *Linguarum sive dictionum exoletarum Hippocratis explicatio.*

Florenz, Bibl. Mediceo Laurentiana, Laurent. plut. 74, 2; s. XI.

(p. 281 b) *De septimestri partu* (Inc. Τῆς κυήσεως οὐχ εἷς ὡρισμένος).

Florenz, Bibl. Mediceo Laurentiana, Laurent. plut. 74, 3; s. XII.

(p. 2) *Adversus Lycum.*
(p. 12) *Adversus ea quae Juliano in Hippocratis aphorismos enuntiata sunt libellus.*
(p. 22) *Linguarum sive dictionum exoletarum Hippocratis explicatio.*
(p. 38) *De optima secta ad Thrasybulum liber.*
(p. 60 b) *De purgantium medicamentorum facultatibus.*
(p. 64 b) *De constitutione artis medicae ad Patrophilum liber.*
(p. 80 b) *De foetuum formatione.*
(p. 91) *An in arteriis natura sanguis contineatur.*
(f. 98) *De instrumento odoratus.*
(p. 98) *De septimestri partu.*
(p. 105 b) *An animal sit quod est in utero.*
(f. 110v) *Thrasybulus sive utrum medicinae sit an gymnastices hygieine.*

(p. 129) *Quod optimus medicus sit etiam philosophus.*
(p. 132) *De optima doctrina.*
(f. 134v) *De parvae pilae exercitatione.*
(p. 136 b) *Quod qualitates incorporeae sint.*
(p. 141 b) *De victus ratione in morbis acutis ex Hippocratis sententia* (Inc. mutil. ἠρεμίαν δὲ καὶ παρηγορίαν. Expl. ἀξιώσομεν).
(p. 149 b) *De cuiuslibet animi peccatorum dignotione atque medela.*
(p. 159 b) *De propriorum animi cuiuslibet affectuum dignotione et curatione.*
(f. 171 b) *De historia philosopha.*
(p. 188 b) *De comate secundum Hippocratem.*
(p. 192) *De motu musculorum libri II* (Pars l. I = K. IV 367–371, 4).

Florenz, Bibl. Mediceo Laurentiana, Laurent. plut. 74, 4; s. c. XII.

(p. 1) *De usu partium corporis humani libri XVII.*

Florenz, Bibl. Mediceo Laurentiana, Laurent. plut. 74, 5; s. XIV.
See also **[plut. 74, (?)]** above (p. 21).

(p. 3) *De elementis secundum Hippocratem.*
(p. 17) *De temperamentis.*
(p. 55) *De facultatibus naturalibus.*
(p. 91) *De substantia facultatum naturalium fragmentum.*
(p. 92 b) *De cuiuslibet animi peccatorum dignotione atque medela.*
(f. 94 b) *De respirationis usu.*
(p. 104) *De praegnotione ad Epigenem.*
(p. 121) *De totius morbi temporibus.*
(p. 123) *De sectis ad eos qui introducuntur.*
(p. 129 b) *De inaequali intemperie.*
(p. 133) *De tumoribus praeter naturam.*
(p. 160) *De theriaca ad Pisonem liber.*
(p. 163) *De antidotis libri II.*
(p. 311) *De pulsibus ad tirones* (Expl. καὶ μαίλακος).

Florenz, Bibl. Mediceo Laurentiana, Laurent. plut. 74, 6; s. XIV.

(p. 1) *Methodi medendi libri XIV.*

Florenz, Bibl. Mediceo Laurentiana, Laurent. plut. 74, 7; s. IX.

(p. 81) *Methodi medendi libri XIV* (Frgm. Lib. VI c. 5–6).
(p. 154) *De machinamentis* (Frgm. Inc. Μόνον μὲν ἱκανόν ἐστι).
(p. 262) *De ossibus ad tirones.*

(f. 286) *De fasciis.*
(p. 312) *In Hippocratis de articulis librum commentarii IV.*

Florenz, Bibl. Mediceo Laurentiana, Laurent. plut. 74, 8; s. XV.

(p. 1) *Hippocratis aphorismi et Galeni in eos commentarii VII.*
(p. 173) *In Hippocratis prognosticum commentarii III.*

Florenz, Bibl. Mediceo Laurentiana, Laurent. plut. 74, 9; s. c. XII.

(p. 1) *De usu partium corporis humani libri XVII.*

Florenz, Bibl. Mediceo Laurentiana, Laurent. plut. 74, 10; s. XIV.

Prognostica (Σημεῖα ἰατρικά etc.).
(p. 13) *De anatomicis administrationibus libri IX* (Frgm. Inc. Ἑκάστῳ τῶν ζώων).
(f. 13v) *De optima corporis nostri constitutione* (Γαλ. περὶ κατασκ. τοῦ ἀνθρώπου. Inc. Οὐ μικρὸν μέν ἐστιν καταφρονῆσαι τὴν Πλάτωνος σοφίαν καὶ Ἀριστοτέλους καὶ Ἀσκληπιάδου καὶ Χείρωνος καὶ Ἱπποκράτους καὶ τοῦ Δημοκρίτου καὶ τοῦ μεγάλου Γαληνοῦ [sic]. Physiologischer Traktat in Frage und Antwort. [M. W.]).
(p. 13 b) *De hominis natura testamentum. De victu singulis mensibus servando* (Frgm. Inc. Οὐ μικρόν μοί ἐστι καταφρονῆσαι).
(p. 82 b) *Remedia* (Varia medicamentorum genera. Inc. Ἐπιμελούμενον τῆς σῆς; *vgl.* Hipp. Ep. ad Ptol.).

Florenz, Bibl. Mediceo Laurentiana, Laurent. plut. 74, 11; s. XIII.

(p. 163) *De typis* (Frgm. Inc. Πολλῶν δὴ πλατύτερον).

Florenz, Bibl. Mediceo Laurentiana, Laurent. plut. 74, 12; s. XV.

(p. 1) *De placitis Hippocratis et Platonis libri IX* (Frgm. Inc. Εἰ γὰρ ἐν τῷ διανοεῖσθαι).
(p. 20) *Methodi medendi libri XIV* (Frgm. ex libb. I. II. VII. IX. XII. XIII).
(p. 26) *De usu partium corporis humani libri XVII* (Excerpta ex libris XI. XIV. XVII).
(p. 28) *De tremore, palpitatione, convulsione et rigore* (brevissimum frgm.).
(p. 28 b) *Galeni in Hippocratis de natura hominis lib. commentarii II* (Frgm.).
(p. 29) *De diebus decretoriis libri III* (Exc. e l. II).
(p. 30) *De elementis secundum Hippocratem* (Excerpta e libro I.).

(p. 30) *De symptomatum causis libri III* (Frgm. e libro II).

Florenz, Bibl. Mediceo Laurentiana, Laurent. plut. 74, 14; s. XV.

(p. 1) *Definitiones medicae.*
(p. 26 b) *Introductio sive medicus.*

Florenz, Bibl. Mediceo Laurentiana, Laurent. plut. 74, 16; s. XIV.

(p. 1) *De differentiis morborum.*
(p. 8 b) *De morborum causis.*
(p. 15 b) *De symptomatum differentiis.*
(f. 19 b) *De symptomatum causis libri III.*
(p. 62) *De locis affectis libri VI* (Διαγνώσεις τόπων πεπονθότων; libri VI).

Florenz, Bibl. Mediceo Laurentiana, Laurent. plut. 74, 17; s. XII.

(p. 133) *De simplicium medicamentorum temperamentis et facultatibus libri XI* (Libri X. XI 1–10).

Florenz, Bibl. Mediceo Laurentiana, Laurent. plut. 74, 18; s. XIV.

(p. 1) *De usu partium corporis humani libri XVII.*
(p. 149) *De dignoscendis pulsibus libri IV.*
(p. 189) *De pulsuum differentiis libri IV.*
(p. 275) *De causis pulsuum libri IV.*
(p. 298 b) *De praesagitione ex pulsibus libri IV.*

Florenz, Bibl. Mediceo Laurentiana, Laurent. plut. 74, 19; s. XIV.
See also **[ap. Bandini III 122]** above (p. 20).

(p. 11) *Ars medica.*

Florenz, Bibl. Mediceo Laurentiana, Laurent. plut. 74, 22; s. XIV.

(p. 1) *De purgantium medicamentorum facultatibus.*
(p. 2 b) *De curandi ratione per venae sectionem.*
(p. 9 b) *De venae sectione* (K. XIX 519–528; des. imperf.).
(p. 15) *De placitis Hippocratis et Platonis libri IX* (Fragmenta libr. II. III. V. VI.).

Florenz, Bibl. Mediceo Laurentiana, Laurent. plut. 74, 25; s. XIV.

(p. 1) *De compositione medicamentorum per genera libri VII.*

(p. 127) *In Hippocratis epidemiarum libros commentarius* (in librum III).
(p. 153) *De probis pravisque alimentorum sucis.*

Florenz, Bibl. Mediceo Laurentiana, Laurent. plut. 74, 28; s. XIV.

(p. 1) *De pulsuum differentiis libri IV.*
(p. 114 b) *De dignoscendis pulsibus libri IV.*
(p. 199 b) *De causis pulsuum libri IV.*
(p. 294 b) *De praesagitione ex pulsibus libri IV.*

Florenz, Bibl. Mediceo Laurentiana, Laurent. plut. 74, 30; s. XIV.

(p. 1) *De locis affectis Libri VI.*

Florenz, Bibl. Mediceo Laurentiana, Laurent. plut. 74, 31; x. XIV.

(p. 22 b) *De urinis* (Inc. Τὴν περὶ τῆς τῶν οὔρων διαφορᾶς).
(p. 199 b) *In Hippocratis prognosticum commentarii III* (Frgm. ex libris I. II. III.).
(f. 206ᵛ) *De pulsuum differentiis libri IV* (Frgm.).
(p. 208) *De typis.*

Florenz, Bibl. Mediceo Laurentiana, Laurent. plut. 75, 5; s. XIV.
»Laurent. 75, 5 + 75, 20 bilden Bd. I, 75, 18 + 75, 7 den II. Bd. derselben Aëtiushandschrift des XIV. Jahrhunderts.« M. W.

(p. 159) *In Hippocratis librum de acutorum victu commentarii IV.*
(p. 249) *In Hippocratis prognosticum commentarii III.*

Florenz, Bibl. Mediceo Laurentiana, Laurent. plut. 75, 7; s. XIV.
»Laurent. 75, 5 + 75, 20 bilden Bd. I, 75, 18 + 75, 7 den II. Bd. derselben Aëtiushandschrift des XIV. Jahrhunderts.« M. W.

(p. 217) *Quos, quibus catharticis medicamentis et quando purgare opporteat.*
(p. 237 b) *De consuetudinibus.*

Florenz, Bibl. Mediceo Laurentiana, Laurent. plut. 75, 8; s. XV.

(p. 9) *De compositione medicamentorum secundum locos libri X.*

Florenz, Bibl. Mediceo Laurentiana, Laurent. plut. 75, 9; s. XV.

(p. 171) *Ad Glauconem de medendi methodo libri II.*

Florenz, Bibl. Mediceo Laurentiana, Laurent. plut. 75, 10; s. XV.

(p. 1) *De succedaneis liber* (Lexicon ordine litterarum compositum, cap. VI tractatus medici anon.).
(p. 1) *Lexicon botanicum* (Cap. V tractatus medici anon.).

Florenz, Bibl. Mediceo Laurentiana, Laurent. plut. 75, 14; s. XV.

(p. 20) *De differentiis febrium libri II.*
(p. 74) *De elementis secundum Hippocratem* (»De quinque sensibus libri II«).

Florenz, Bibl. Mediceo Laurentiana, Laurent. plut. 75, 16; s. XV.

(p. 148 b) *Ad Glauconem de medendi methodo libri II.*

Florenz, Bibl. Mediceo Laurentiana, Laurent. plut. 75, 17; s. XIV.

(p. 1) *Remedia* (Quaedam remedia evacuantia. Inc. Τοῖς ἀποδακρυτικοῖς χρώμεθα).
(p. 4) *De compositione medicamentorum secundum locos libri X.*

Florenz, Bibl. Mediceo Laurentiana, Laurent. plut. 75, 19; s. XIV.

(p. 12) *De urinis.*
(p. 193) *De vita et morte.*

Florenz, Bibl. Mediceo Laurentiana, Laurent. App., 2; s. XV.
= Antinori 101 (*Census*: 80, nr [0372]).

(f. –) *De angina.*
(f. 222) **Hippokrates**, **Galenos**, *Jatrosophium* (Ἰατρικὸν Ἱππ. καὶ Γαλ. ἰατρεῖαι διάφοροι).
(f. 344) *De iecore.*
(f. 359) *Fauces definiuntur.*

Florenz, Magliabech.
Now Firenze, Biblioteca nazionale Magliabechiana

Florenz, Magliabech. 1; s. XVI.

(f. 207v) *De urinis* (Inc. Τί δηλοῖ τὸ λεπτὸν καὶ ὠχρὸν οὖρον. Expl. τοῦ μελαγχολικοῦ χυμοῦ).

Florenz, Bibl. Riccardiana
Firenze, Biblioteca Riccardiana

Florenz, Bibl. Riccardiana, Riccard. 17 (K I 24); s. XVI.
Now Riccard. 17 (*Census*: 81, nr [0378]).

(f. 111) *In Hippocratis prognosticum commentarii III.*

Florenz, Bibl. Riccardiana, Riccard. 41 (K II 2); XVI.
Now Riccard. 41 (*Census*: 81, nr [0380]).

(f. 13) *De urinis ex Hippocrate, Galeno aliisque quibusdam.*

Florenz, Bibl. Riccardiana, Riccard. 44 (K II 5); s. XV–XVI.
Now Riccard. 44 (*Census*: 81, nr [0381]).

(f. 27) *Hippocratis aphorismi et Galeni in eos commentarii VII.*
(f. 192) *In Hippocratis prognosticum commentarii III.*
(f. 242) *De dignotione ex insomniis.*
(f. 243^{v}) *De praenotione.*

Genf

Genf, Genev. Bibl. Urb., 42; s. XVI.
Genève, Bibliothèque de Genève, MS grec 42 (*Census*: 83, nr [0385]).

(f. 1) *De simplicium medicamentorum temperamentis et facultatibus libri XI.*

Grottaferrata

Grottaferrata, Klosterbibliothek, 2 Γ VI (series IX cod. 46); s. XIV.
Now Biblioteca del Monumento nazionale di Grottaferrata, Z.γ.VI (GR 81) (*Census*: 86, nr [0395]).

(f. 1) *De ossibus ad tirones.*
(f. 18) *De musculorum dissectione.*
(f. 50) *De venarum arteriarumque dissectione.*
(f. 58) *De nervorum dissectione.*

Jena, Universitätsbibliothek.
Now Thüringer Universitäts- und Landesbibliothek

Jena, Universitätsbibliothek, Aldina c. nott. Cornarii.

Opera varia.

Jerusalem, Bibl. d. hl. Grabes
Now at Αθήνα, Εθνική Βιβλιοθήκη της Ελλάδος ΕΒΕ, Μετόχιον Παναγίου Τάφου–ΜΠΤ

Jerusalem, Bibl. d. hl. Grabes, 179; s. XV.
Now ΜΠΤ 179 (*Census*: 92, nr [0410] and p. 15).

(f. 202) *De morbis Excerpta* (Σύντομος διδασκαλία Γαλ. τοῦ σπεύσαντος γράψαι εἰς τὰ τῶν μορίων πάθη κτλ.).

Jerusalem, Bibl. d. hl. Grabes, 199; s. –.
Now ΜΠΤ 199 (*Census*: 92, nr [0412] and p. 15).

(f. 64 A) *De hominis natura testamentum. De victu singulis mensibus servando* (Δίαιτα ἀκριβὴς π. τῶν τεσσάρ. στοιχείων τοῦ χρόνου καὶ περὶ καταστάσεως ὑγιεινῆς τοῦ ἀνθρώπου καὶ τῆς κατασκευῆς αὐτοῦ).

Jerusalem, Bibl. d. hl. Grabes, 363; a. 1596.
Now ΜΠΤ 363 (*Census*: 92, nr [0416] and p. 15).

(f. 211 B) *De hominis natura testamentum. De victu singulis mensibus servando* (*Wie* nr. 199 [= Jerusalem, Bibl, d. hl. Grabes 199] above).

Jerusalem, Bibl. d. Hl. Kreuzes

Jerusalem, Bibl. d. Hl. Kreuzes, 68; s. –.
= Πατριαρχείο 68 (*Census*: 93, nr [0418]).
(*Census*: 93, nr [0418]).

(nr 2) *De hominis natura testamentum. De victu singulis mensibus servando* (*Wie im* Athous Διονυσ. [3701. 167] [above p. 6]).

Jerusalem, Bibl. d. Hl. Kreuzes, 85; s. XVI.
= Ιερά Μονή Τιμίου Σταυρού, 85 (*Census*: 93, nr [0419]).

(f. 165) *Excerpta varia* (Πῶς γράφονται αἱ εἰκόνες Ὁμήρου ... Γαληνοῦ ...).

Jerusalem, Bibl. Mar-Saba
Ιερουσαλήμ, Πατριαρχείο, Ιερά Μονή Αγίου Σάββα

Jerusalem, Bibl. Mar-Saba, 432; a. 1662.
= Ιερά Μονή Αγίου Σάββα, 432 (*Census*: 93, nr [0421]).

(f. 1) **Hippokrates, Galenos, Meletius monachus,** *Jatrosophium* (Ἰατροσόφιον ... Γαλ. Ἱππ. καὶ Μελετίου).

Jerusalem, Bibl. Mar-Saba, 481; s. XVIII.
= Ιερά Μονή Αγίου Σάββα, 481 (*Census*: 93, nr [0422]).

(f. 265) *Hippocratis aphorismi et Galeni in eos commentarii VII* (Μετάφρασις τῶν ἀφ. τοῦ Ἱππ. εἰς τὴν κοινὴν διάλεκτον ... ἐκ τῆς τοῦ Γαλ. διδασκαλίας).

Jerusalem, Bibl. patriarch.
Ιερουσαλήμ, Πατριαρχείο, Πανάγιος Τάφος

Jerusalem, Bibl. patriarch., 102; s. XVIII.
= Πανάγιος Τάφος, 102 (*Census*: 94, nr [0425]).

(f. 12) *Hippocratis aphorismi et Galeni in eos commentarii VII* (Ἑρμηνεία εἰς τοὺς ἀφ. Ἱππ., καταστρωθεῖσα εἰς κοινὴν φράσιν παρὰ Μπαλάνου Βασιλοπούλου ... κατὰ τὸν Γαληνόν).

Jerusalem, Bibl. patriarch., 148; s. XVI.
= Πανάγιος Τάφος, 148 (*Census*: 94, nr [0427]).

(f. 4) *De humoribus* (Π. στοιχ. κ. χυμ. Inc. Ὁ κόσμος οὗτος).
(f. 40) *De unguentis* (Π. ἀλ. ἐκ τοῦ Ἱππ. καὶ Γαλ. καὶ ἑτέρων φιλοσ. κ. ἰατρ.).

Kopenhagen, Bibl. Univ.
Now København, Kongelige Bibliotek

Kopenhagen, Bibl. Univ., e donatione variorum 4° 42; s. XVI.
Now e don. var. 42, 4° (*Census*: 102, nr [0448]).
See also **Padua, Bibl. Joann. Rhodii** below (p. 59).

Ars medica.

Kopenhagen, Bibl. Univ., e donatione variorum Fol. 14; s. XV–XVI.
Now e don. var. 14, 2° (*Census*: 102, nr [0450]).

(f. 1) *Synopsis librorum suorum sedecim de pulsibus.*

Kopenhagen, Königl. Bibliothek
Now København, Det Kongelige Bibliotek

Kopenhagen, Königl. Bibliothek, Hauniens. ant. fund. reg. 224; s. XVI.
Now GkS 224, 2° (*Census*: 102, nr [0445]).

Linguarum sive dictionum exoletarum Hippocratis explicatio.

Kopenhagen, Königl. Bibliothek, Hauniens. ant. fund. reg. 225; s. XVI.
Now GkS 225, 2° (*Census*: 102, nr [0446]).

Excerpta varia (Frgm. Inc. μηδ' ὅλως δάκνοντα. Expl. ῥοδόσταγμα καὶ οἶνος).
(f. 1) *De anatomicis administrationibus libri IX.*
(f. 176) *De compositione medicamentorum per genera libri VII* (Inc. wie im Berol. Phillipps. [1529] [above p. 11]. Expl. = K. XIII 1058).
(f. 114) *De antidotis libri II* (Expl. mutil. καὶ οὕτω λοιπὸν ἀκριβῶς).
(f. 170) *De theriaca ad Pisonem liber.*

Kopenhagen, Königl. Bibliothek, Hauniens. ant. fund. reg. 1648; s. XV.
Now GkS 1648, 4° (*Census*: 102, nr [0447]).

Definitiones medicae.

Leipzig

Leipzig, Institut f. Geschichte der Medizin, Basileensis (1538) des Galen.
Now Leipzig, Universitätabibliothek, Sudhoff III 815 a–e (*Census*: 106, nr [0453]).

Basileensis (1538) des Galen mit Varianten und Korrekturen von der Hand des Leo Allatius.).

Leipzig, Universitätsbibliothek
Now Leipzig, Universitätsbibliothek «Bibliotheca Albertina»

Leipzig, Universitätsbibliothek, 50; s. XVI.
= Cod. graec. 50 (*Census*: 106, nr [0454]).

(f. 1) *De locis affectis Libri VI.*
(f. 132) *De sanitate tuenda Libri VI.*

Leipzig, Universitätsbibliothek, 51; s. –.
= Cod. graec. 51 (*Census*: 106, nr [0455]).

(f. 1) *De symptomatum causis libri III* (Libri I et II).
(f. 41) *De simplicium medicamentorum temperamentis et facultatibus libri XI.*

Leipzig, Universitätsbibliothek, 52; s. XVI.
= Cod. graec. 52 (*Census*: 106, nr [0456]).

(f. 1) *Introductio sive medicus.*
(f. 40) *Definitiones medicae.*
(f. 57) *De anatomicis administrationibus libri IX.*

Leipzig, Universitätsbibliothek, 54; s. XIX.
= Cod. graec. 54 (*Census*: 107, nr [0458]).

De musculorum dissectione.

Leipzig, Universitätsbibliothek, 55; a. 1561.
= Cod. graec. 55 (*Census*: 107, nr [0459]).

Ars medica.

Leipzig, Universitätsbibliothek, 56; s. XIX.
= Cod. graec. 56 (*Census*: 107, nr [0460]).

In Hippocratis de humoribus librum commentarii III.

Leipzig, Universitätsbibliothek, 57; s. XVIII–XIX.
= Cod. graec. 57 (*Census*: 107, nr [0461]).

Opera varia (»Vier gelbe Pappbände: Jo. Scaligeri emendatt. in Gal. ex exemplo Guelferbyt. I–IV. Am Schluß 2 lose Hefte eingelegt, das eine d. d. 15. Juli 1616: In Gal. libellum qui inscr. π. ὀστῶν«).
Excerpta varia (Jo. Scaligeri emendatt. in Gal. ex exemplo Guelferbyt. I–IV).

Leipzig, Universitätsbibliothek, 58; s. XVI (?).
= Cod. graec. 58 (*Census*: 107, nr [0462]).

Opera varia (»Cornarius in Galenum. Coniecturae Cornarii excerptae ex Aldinae editionis exemplo in bibl. Jenensi asservato«. *Vgl. oben* Jena).

Lesbos, Βιβλ. τῆς τοῦ Λειμῶνος Μονῆς
Now Καλλονή Λέσβου, Βιβλιοθήκη τῆς τοῦ Λειμῶνος Μονῆς

Lesbos, Βιβλ. τῆς τοῦ Λειμῶνος Μονῆς, 175; s. XVII.
Καλλονή Λέσβου, Βιβλιοθήκη τῆς τοῦ Λειμῶνος Μονῆς, 175.

Excerpta varia.

Leyden, Universitäts-Bibliothek
Now Leiden, Universiteitsbibliotheek

Leyden, Universitäts-Bibliothek, B. P., 2 A; s. XVI.
= Bibliotheca Publica Graeca 2 A (now BPG 2 A) (*Census*: 109, nr [0475]).

Ad Glauconem de medendi methodo libri II (e Steph. interpr. Lib. I).

Leyden, Universitäts-Bibliothek, B. P., 16; s. XV.
= Bibliotheca Publica Graeca 16 (now BPG 16) (*Census*: 109, nr [0477]).

De simplicium medicamentorum temperamentis et facultatibus libri XI.

Leyden, Universitäts-Bibliothek, Miscell. 11; s. XIII.
= *Vossianus miscellaneus* 11 (now VMI 11) (*Census*: 115, nr [0518]).

(f. 29–44) *Ad Glauconem de medendi methodo libri II* (*Vielleicht zur* Θεραπ. μέθοδ. *gehörig*).
(f. 29–44) *Methodi medendi libri XIV* (Init. et fine mutil.; fort. Therapeut. ad Glauconem).

Leyden, Universitäts-Bibliothek, Scalig. 18; s. XVI.
= *Scaligerianus* 18 (now SCA 18) (*Census*: 110, nr [0482]).
See also **Scalig. 18?** below.

De elementis secundum Hippocratem.
De facultatibus naturalibus.
De morborum causis.
De symptomatum causis libri III.
De symptomatum differentiis.
De temperamentis.

Leyden, Universitäts-Bibliothek, Scalig. 18?; s. XVI.
Same as **Scalig. 18** above (*Census*: 110, nr [0483]).
= *Scaligerianus* 18 (now SCA 18).

De differentiis morborum.

[Leyden, Universitäts-Bibliothek, Vossian. ?; s. –].
= *Vossianus graecus* in folio 11 (now VGF 11) (*Census*: 110, nr [0487]).
See **Voss. fol. 11** below (p. 35).

De symptomatum differentiis.

[Leyden, Universitäts-Bibliothek, Vossian. ?].
= *Vossianus graecus* in folio 53 (now VGF 53) (*Census*: 110, nr [0488]).
See **Voss. fol. 53** below (p. 35).

Methodi medendi libri XIVI (in. et fin. mut.).

[Leyden, Universitäts-Bibliothek, Voss. Cat. bibl. Lugd. Bat. p. 398 n. 50].
= *Vossianus graecus* in quarto 50 (now VGQ 50) (*Census*: 111, nr [0489]).

Hippiatrosophium.

[Leyden, Universitäts-Bibliothek, Voss. 16; s. –].
= *Vossianus graecus* in quarto 17 (now VGQ 17) (*Census*: 111, nr [0491]).
See **Voss. 4° 17** below.

Ars medica.

[Leyden, Universitäts-Bibliothek, Voss. 31; s. –].
= *Vossianus graecus* in folio 31 (now VGF 31) (*Census*: 111, nr [0493]).

De urinis.

[Leyden, Universitäts-Bibliothek, Vossian. 58].
= *Vossianus graecus* in folio 58 (now VGF 58) (*Census*: 111, nr [0494]).

De theriaca ad Pisonem liber.

[Leyden, Universitäts-Bibliothek, Voss. 2168; s. –].
= *Vossianus graecus* in folio 59 (now VGF 59) (*Census*: 111–112, nr [0495]).

De pulsuum differentiis libri IV.

[Leyden, Universitäts-Bibliothek, Vossian. 2324].
= *Vossianus graecus* in folio 10 (now VGF 10^{I}, 10^{II}, 10^{III}) (*Census*: 112, nr [0496]).

De septimestri partu.

Leyden, Universitäts-Bibliothek, Voss. 4° 17; s. XV.
= *Vossianus graecus* in quarto 17 (now VGQ 17) (*Census*: 113, nr [0498]).
See also **[Voss. 16]** above.

Ars medica.

Leyden, Universitäts-Bibliothek, Voss. 4° 45; s. XIV.
= *Vossianus graecus* in quarto 45 (now VGQ 45) (*Census*: 113, nr [0500]).

De crisibus libri III.
De differentiis morborum.
De dignotione ex insomniis.
De praenotione.
De venae sectione (K. XIX 519–528).
Quomodo morbum simulantes sint deprehendi.
Quos, quibus catharticis medicamentis et quando purgare opporteat.

Leyden, Universitäts-Bibliothek, Voss. fol. 11; s. XVI.
= *Vossianus graecus* in folio 11 (now VGF 11) (*Census*: 113, nr [0507]).
See also [**Vossian.** ?] above (p. 33).

De symptomatum causis libri III.

Leyden, Universitäts-Bibliothek, Voss. fol. 27; s. XVI.
= *Vossianus graecus* in folio 27 (now VGF 27) (*Census*: 114, nr [0510]).

De anatomicis administrationibus libri IX (Frgm. Anatomica; non integrum opus. Expl. ὅλον ἐγκεφάλου τὸ καλούμενον ὑπό τινων).

Leyden, Universitäts-Bibliothek, Voss. fol. 53; s. XV.
= *Vossianus graecus* in folio 53 (now VGF 53) (*Census*: 114, nr [0513]).
See also [**Vossian.** ?] above (p. 33).

Ad Glauconem de medendi methodo libri II.
De locis affectis libri VI (Περὶ διαγνώσεως τ. πεπ. τόπ.).

Leyden, Universitäts-Bibliothek, Voss. Miscell. 1 pars 13; s. XV.
= *Vossianus miscellaneus* 1 (now VMI 1) (*Census*: 114–115, nr [0517]).

Linguarum sive dictionum exoletarum Hippocratis explicatio.

Leyden, Universitäts-Bibliothek, Vulc. 43; s. XV.
= *Vulcanianus* 43 (now VUL 43) (*Census*: 115, nr [0520]).

De causis pulsuum libri IV.
De dignoscendis pulsibus libri IV.
De praesagitione ex pulsibus libri IV.
De pulsuum differentiis libri IV.

Leyden, Universitäts-Bibliothek, Vulc. 57; s. XVI.
= *Vulcanianus* 57 (now VUL 57) (*Census*: 115, nr [0522]).

De anatomicis administrationibus libri IX (Expl. [l. IV] τῷ δ' ὑποτεταμένῳ τῷ μετὰ τὸ μέτωπον δέρματι μυώδη φύσιν ἐγνώκασι μὲν οἱ περὶ τὰς ἀνα ...).

London, British Museum
Now London, British Library

London, British Museum, Addit. 6898; s. XIII (XIV), XIII/XIV.
See also **Venedig, Monast. S. Michaelis prope Murianum, 93** below (p. 102).

(f. 1) *Methodi medendi libri XIV.*
Hippokrates: (f. 160^{v}) *Aphorismi* (c. scholiis; Inc. ⟨ἐπε⟩ιδή⟨π⟩ερ ἐνταῦθα σκοπὸν ἔχει ὁ Γαληνός).

London, British Museum, Addit. 10, 058; s. XV.

(f. 58^{v}) *De succedaneis liber* (Inc. Ἀντὶ ἀκανθίου = K. XIX 723. Expl. Ἀντὶ βαλσαμελαίου κτλ. deest ap. K.).
(f. 65) *Remedia* (Σκευασία τῆς ἱερᾶς).
(f. 71^{v}) *De hominis natura testamentum. De victu singulis mensibus servando* (*Wie im* Athous Ἰβήρων [5034. 914] [above p. 8]. Expl. καλῶς χρωμένοις, καὶ παραφυλάττουσι ταῦτα).
(f. 74) *Remedia* (Δυναμερόν. Inc. Ὁ περὶ τῶν ἀντιδότων καὶ ἐλαίων. Expl. καρποβαλσάμου κόκκους κ', νάμ · [sic !] ταύρων).
(f. 106^{v}) *Remedia* (Περὶ ἐλαίων καὶ μύρων. Inc. Ὀμφάκινον ἔλαιον γίνεται. Expl. καὶ βράσας ἕως συστάσεως ἔχει πολυτίμως).
(f. 115^{v}) *Remedia* (Περὶ ἁπλῶν διδομένων φαρμάκων. Inc. Ἐλατήριον · καθαίρει φλέγμα καὶ χολὴν ὅσον. Expl. καὶ ὀλίγον οἶνον ὕδωρ ἄγει).
(f. 123) *Remedia* (Sine auctoris nomine. Περὶ συνθέτων φαρμάκων καὶ τίσι ταῦτα δοτέον. Inc. Τὸ διακιτρίου [sic !] καθαίρει μὲν φλέγμα. Expl. πρόσβαλλε δακρύ^{δ} κεράτια δ').
(f. 127) *De dignotione hominum purgandorum.*
(f. 128) *Remedia* (Περὶ δυνάμεων ἐμπλάστρων. Inc. Ἡ διάμπαρος τονοῖ καταπαν^{τ} [sic]. Expl. [?] βράσας τὸ ἀφέψημα ἄντλιε).

London, British Museum, Addit. 11, 888; s. XV.

(f. 1) *Definitiones medicae.*
(f. 25) *De usu partium corporis humani libri XVII* (In fine epigr. inc. ἥδε βίβλος σύμπασα. expl. πλέξε φύσηϊ Θεός).

London, British Museum, Addit. 17, 900; s. XVII.

(f. 93) *De urinis* (Inc. Οὖρον λευκόν).
(f. 204^{v}) *De venae sectione* (Inc. Οἱ πρῶτοι καὶ κυριώτατοι σκοποί. Expl. καὶ ταῦτα μὲν ἐπιεικεῖ [?] φάρμακον).
(f. 272) *De venae sectione* (Inc. *wie auf f.* 204^{v}. Expl. εἰ γὰρ πλησιάσει τούτῳ).

London, British Museum, Addit. 28, 830; s. XVII.

(f. 15) *Iatrosophia* (Ἰ. … ἐκ τῶν βιβλίων τοῦ Ἱππ. καὶ Γαλ.).

London, British Museum, Arundelian.; s. XV in.
= Arundel 537 (*Census*: 118, nr [0536]).

(f. 114) *Ad Glauconem de medendi methodo libri II.*

London, British Museum, Burneian. 94; s. XV–XVI, XV (XVI).

(f. 170) *De cerebro.*

London, British Museum, Burneian. 523; s. XVIII.

(f. 9) *Opera varia* (»Emendationes in quosdam Galeni locos ed. Basil. 1538 manu Ant. Askew scriptae«).

London, British Museum, Harleian. 5611; s. XV.

(f. 1) *Hippocratis aphorismi et Galeni in eos commentarii VII.*

London, British Museum, Harleian. 5625; s. XV (XVI).

(f. 1) *De pulsuum differentiis libri IV.*
(f. 91) *De dignoscendis pulsibus libri IV.*
(f. 157) *De causis pulsuum libri IV* (Inscr. περὶ αἰτίων τῶν σφυγμῶν).
(f. 226) *De praesagitione ex pulsibus libri IV.*

London, British Museum, Harleian. 5626; s. XV (XVI), XV (XVI ?), XV–XVI, XV–XVI (?).

(f. 2) **Hippokrates**, **Galenos**, *Jatrosophium* (Ἰατροσόφ. … Ἱππ. καὶ Γαλ. κτλ.).
(f. 53) *De victus ratione* (Διαιτητικὸν ὑγιεινῶν παραγγελμάτων).
(f. 53v) *De sanitate tuenda libri VI* (Frgm. Ἐκ τῶν ὑγιεινῶν τοῦ Γαλ. προοίμιον, τί ἐστιν ὑγεία καὶ τίνες οἱ ἄριστα κατεσκευασμένοι. Inc. Τῆς περὶ τὸ σῶμα κτλ. Expl. δίαιτα λεπτύνουσα καὶ χρίσματα μετρίως θερμαίνοντα).

London, British Museum, Harleian. 5651; s. XV–XVI.

De locis affectis Libri VI (c. scholiis).

London, British Museum, Harleian. 5652; s. XV, XVI.

De usu partium corporis humani libri XVII (*Am Schlusse dasselbe Epigr. wie im* [Londin.] Addit. 11, 888 [above p. 36]).

London, British Museum, Harleian. 6305; s. XVI, XVI (?).

(f. 6) *De crisibus libri III.*
(f. 83) *De diebus decretoriis libri III.*
(f. 153) *Lexicon botanicum* (Inc. *und* Expl *wie im* Berolin. [Phill. 1570] [above p. 11]).

London, British Museum, Regius 16 C XI; s. XVI.
Now Royal. 16.C.xi (*Census*: 120, nr [0555]).

(f. 1) *De diebus decretoriis libri III.*

London, Medical Society
Now at the Wellcome Library, London

London, Medical Society, –.
Now London, Wellcome Library, MS. MSL 83 (*Census*: 121, nr [0561]).

Indices in Galenum (»nicht aufzufinden«. Kalbfl. *Vgl.* Costomiris Revue des études grecques II [1889] p. 381. Index auctorum a Gal. citatorum).

London, Medical Society, HHi 17 = We 30; s. XV in.
Now London, Wellcome Library, MS. MSL 60 (*Census*: 121, nr [0564]).

Remedia.
(f. 56) *De ponderibus et mensuris* (Inscr. Περὶ σταθμῶν Γαληνοῦ. Inc. Ὁ σταθμὸς βάρει μετρούμενος. Expl. ἄποιόν ἐστι κατὰ τὴν διαφοράν).
(nr 27 Dbg.) *De urinis.*
(nr 33 Dbg.) *De excrementis* (Expl. τὸ ἧπορ αὐτοῦ βεβλαμμένον).
(nr 37 Dbg.) *De pulsibus* (Inc. Ὁ σφυγμὸς κίνησίς ἐστιν. Expl. εἰς τὸ βάθος τοῦ σώματος, ὕστερον δέ. Daremberg, Mscrts. méd. de l'Angleterre I 162: »apocryphe«).
(nr 40 Dbg.) *De remediis parabilibus libri III* (Liber I. Expl. θαυμάσεις δὲ πάνυ δεξάμενος · τῶν εὐπορίστων ἰαμάτων δὴ πέρας).

London, Medical Society, HH i 21. 22 = We 28. 29; s. XV.
Now London, Wellcome Library, MS. MSL 52 A&B (*Census*: 121, nr [0565]).

(f. 333^v^) *De pulsibus* (Inc. Αἴσθησιν ἐναρμονίῳ τινὶ κινήσει. Expl. βραδὺς πυκνὸς ἀραιὸς καὶ ἀνώμαλος).
(f. 341) *De pulsibus* (Inc. *wie im* [London Medical Society] H Hi 17 [above]. Expl. ἐπεὶ πολλάκις καὶ παραυτίκα τελευτᾷ).

Madrid, Nationalbibliothek
Madrid, Biblioteca Nacional

Madrid, Nationalbibliothek, 4631 (N 110); a. 1474.
= 4631 (*Census*: 125, nr [0579]).

(f. 155) *De lapidibus* (Inscr. Π. λίθων Διοσκορίδου. »Hic commentarius apud Iriarte impressus ex Dioscuride Aëtio Galeno aliis consutus est«).

Madrid, Nationalbibliothek, 4783 (olim O 67); s. XVI.
= 4783 (*Census*: 126, nr [0584]).

(f. 30) *Prognostica de decubitu ex mathematica scientia*.

Madrid, Bibliothek des Königs

Madrid, Privatbibliothek des Königs, 44 (olim 23); s. XV ex.
Now Salamanca, Biblioteca universitaria, 2659 (*Census*: 127, nr [0589]).

(f. 180^v^) *De theriaca* (π. τῆς μεγάλης θηριακῆς τῆς δι' ἐχιδνῶν. Inc. Πολλῆς οὔσης διαφωνίας περὶ τὰς γραφικὰς ἀποδείξεις. Expl. δεῖ δὲ σαρκῶν μὲν δύο μέρη βάλλεσθαι, ἄρτων δὲ ἕν).

Mailand, Archivio del Capitolo Metropolitano
Milano, Archivio del Capitolo Metropolitano

Mailand, Arch. del Capitolo Metropolitano, 2; s. XV.
= Milano, Archivio del Capitolo Metropolitano, II, E 2, 17 (*Census*: 128, nr [0590]).

(f. 132^v^–135) *Lexicon botanicum* (Inc. *und* Expl. *wie im* Berol. [Phill. 1570] [above p. 11]).

Mailand, Bibl. Ambrosiana
Milano, Biblioteca Ambrosiana

Mailand, Bibl. Ambrosiana, A 45 Sup.; s. XIII.

(f. 31ᵛ) *De lapidibus.*
(f. 43ᵛ) *De alimentorum facultatibus libri III.*

Mailand, Bibl. Ambrosiana, A 80 Sup.; s. XV ex.

(f. 261ᵛ) *Excerpta varia.*

Mailand, Bibl. Ambrosiana, A 95 Sup.; s. XV.

(f. 78) *De morbis Excerpta.*
(f. 78, 91) *Excerpta varia.*

Mailand, Bibl. Ambrosiana, A 156 Sup.; s. XVI.

(f. 24) *Hippocratis aphorismi et Galeni in eos commentarii VII.*
(f. 190) *In Hippocratis prognosticum commentarii III.*
(f. 263) *De dignotione ex insomniis.*
(f. 264) *De praenotione.*

Mailand, Bibl. Ambrosiana, B 90 Sup.; s. XVI.

Definitiones medicae.

Mailand, Bibl. Ambrosiana, B 108 Sup.; s. XIV in.

(f. 19 [fals. pro f. 35; vid. Infra]) *De alimentorum facultatibus libri III* (Libri III = K. VI. VI 533, 9–745, 15/16).
(f. 35) *De alimentorum facultatibus libri III.*
(f. 128) *De venae sectione adversus Erasistrateos Romae degentes* (= K. XI 222–249).
(f. 140) *De venae sectione adversus Erasistratum.*
(f. 158ᵛ) *De curandi ratione per venae sectionem.*
(f. 185) *De theriaca ad Pamphilianum* (Expl. K. XIV 306, 11).

Mailand, Bibl. Ambrosiana, B 126 Sup.; s. XIV, XIV ex.

(f. 130) *De remediis parabilibus libri III* (»Liber II = K. XIV 391 et 383, 4–6«).

Mailand, Bibl. Ambrosiana, B 157 Sup.; s. XV–XVI.

(f. 133) *De aquis* (Inc. καὶ λάπαρα τῶν ἄλλων ἁπάντων ὑδάτων. Galeni esse frgm. putat Schoene).

Mailand, Bibl. Ambrosiana, C 4 Sup.; s. –, XV.

(f. 222) *De uteri dissectione* (»Lacunae crebrae intercapedinibus indicatae sunt«).
(f. 233) *Puero epileptico consilium*.
(f. 244[v]) *De venae sectione* (Inc. *wie im Londinens.* [Brit. Mus. Addit. 17, 900] [above p. 36]).

Mailand, Bibl. Ambrosiana, C 102 Sup.; s. XV.
See also **C 102 Inf.** below (p. 44).

(f. 128) *Ars medica* (not C 102 Inf.).

Mailand, Bibl. Ambrosiana, C 118 Sup.; s. –.
Ambros. muß heißen C 119 Sup.; s. XVI.
See **C 119 Sup.** below.

In Hippocratis de humoribus librum commentarii III (non sine lacunis, ut videtur).

Mailand, Bibl. Ambrosiana, C 119 Sup.; s. XV.
= *L 119 sup. and not C 119 sup.*
= **L 119 Sup**. See also **C 118 Sup.** above.

In Hippocratis de humoribus librum commentarii III.

Mailand, Bibl. Ambrosiana, C 120 Sup.; s. XVI in.

(f. 69 *und* 109) *Synopsis librorum suorum sedecim de pulsibus* (*zweimal in ders. Hds.*).

Mailand, Bibl. Ambrosiana, E 6 Sup.; s. XIII.

(f. 235) *Excerpta varia* (Inc. Τὴν γὰρ λογικὴν παρὰ τοῖς φιλοσόφοις. Expl. τῶν γε γραμμάτων μνημονεύειν δυνάμενον).

Mailand, Bibl. Ambrosiana, E 37 Sup.; s. XVI.

(f. 278) *De succedaneis liber*.

Mailand, Bibl. Ambrosiana, E 105 Sup.; s. –, XIII.

De simplicium medicamentorum temperamentis et facultatibus libri XI (A lib. I–V ἐναντίως ἔχειν σπέρματα τὴν δ' αὐ...).

Mailand, Bibl. Ambrosiana, F 112 Sup.; XV.

(f. 1) *De symptomatum differentiis.*
(f. 15v) *De symptomatum causis libri III* (In margine emendationes et variae lectiones).

Mailand, Bibl. Ambrosiana, G 97 Sup.; s. XVI (XV).

(f. 1) *De differentiis morborum* (Frgm.).
(f. 8) *De morborum causis* (Frgm.).
(f. 15) *De symptomatum differentiis* (Frgm.).
(f. 22) *De symptomatum causis libri III* (Frgm.).
(f. 56) *Ars medica* (Inc. Εἴρηται μὲν οὖν. Expl. βιβλία ἐπιγραφὴν ἔχοντα).
(f. 57) *Methodi medendi libri XIV* (Frgm. Τῆς μεγάλης θεραπευτικῆς λόγος α'. Inc. Τολμηρότατε Θεσσαλέ. Expl. ἐν μὲν δὴ τοῖς τοιούτοις ἅπασι προ... Esse excerptum hoc opus conicit Schoene).

Mailand, Bibl. Ambrosiana, O 50 Sup.; s. –.
s. XIII ex.

De pulsuum differentiis libri IV (Libri IV; fine mutil. Expl. σαφηνίζεσθαι καὶ μὴ κεναῖς ὕπονοι ...).
(f. 129v) *De dignoscendis pulsibus libri IV.*

Mailand, Bibl. Ambrosiana, O 117 Sup.; s. –.
s. XV–XVI.

(f. 89) *De hominis natura testamentum. De victu singulis mensibus servando* (*Wie im* Hierosol. Bibl. d. hl. Grabes 199 [above p. 28]).

Mailand, Bibl. Ambrosiana, P 90 Sup.; s. XV–XVI.

(f. 68) *De corporis partibus* (Inscr. Ὀνομασίαι τῶν ἐκτὸς τοῦ σώματος μορίων. Inc. Πρῶτον μὲν Ἀριστοτέλης. Expl. ἢ ἐκ τῆς κατὰ τὴν θέσιν τάξεως).

Mailand, Bibl. Ambrosiana, Q 3 Sup.; s. XV–XVI.

De symptomatum causis libri III.
(f. 1) *De symptomatum differentiis.*

(f. 45) *De locis affectis libri VI.*
(f. 129) *In Hippocratis praedictionum librum primum commentarii III.*
(f. 185) *De propriis placitis* (Frgm.).
(f. 185^{v}) *De substantia facultatum naturalium fragmentum* (Inc. ὥσπερ ὅτι ψυχὴν ἔχομεν = K. IV 760, 3. Subscr. *als Titel* Περὶ τῶν ἑαυτῷ δοκούντων).
(f. 187) *De libris propriis.*
(f. 197) *De ordine librorum suorum ad Eugenianum.*
(f. 200) *De parvae pilae exercitatione.*
(f. 202^{v}) *Quod qualitates incorporeae sint.*
(f. 207^{v}) *De captionibus penes dictionem.*
(f. 212) *De periodis.*
(f. 225) *De purgantium medicamentorum facultatibus.*
(f. 231) *De atra bile.*
(f. 238) *De plenitudine.*
(f. 265) *De praegnotione ad Epigenem.*

Mailand, Bibl. Ambrosiana, Q 52 Sup.; s. –, XIV.

De locis affectis libri VI (= K. VIII 97–376. Expl. πρὸς αὐτὰ τὸ αἷμα καὶ τὴν ὀρεκτικὴν τῶν).

Mailand, Bibl. Ambrosiana, Q 87 Sup.; s. –.
s. XIV–XV, XV.

(f. 222) *De ossibus ad tirones.*
(f. 222) *Excerpta varia* (Exc. De ossibus et musculis).
(f. 222) *De musculorum dissectione* (Frgm.).

Mailand, Bibl. Ambrosiana, Q 94 Sup.; s. –.
s. XV–XVI.

(f. 8^{v}) *De remediis parabilibus libri III* (Liber II. Inc. Ἐπιζητήσαντός μου. Expl. καὶ καταχρασθὲν ἐπιτιθέμενον).
(f. 29^{v}) *De diebus decretoriis libri III.*
(f. 332) *De urinis* (Inc. Οὖρον λευκὸν μὴ ἔχον ὑπόστασιν).

Mailand, Bibl. Ambrosiana, S 3 Sup.; s. –, XV ex–XVI in, XVI.
s. XV/XVI, XV–XVI.

De ossibus ad tirones.

Mailand, Bibl. Ambrosiana, T 19 Sup.; s. –.
s. XV.

(f. 22) *Definitiones medicae.*

Mailand, Bibl. Ambrosiana, A 81 Inf.; s. –.
s. XIII ex.

(f. 1) *De simplicium medicamentorum temperamentis et facultatibus libri XI* (A lib. V 2 usque ad l. IX in. πόλιν ἐκείνην τῆς μυρί...).

Mailand, Bibl. Ambrosiana, C 80 Inf.; s. –, XVI.

(f. 1) *De anatomicis administrationibus libri IX.*

Mailand, Bibl. Ambrosiana, C 102 Inf.; s. –, XV.
nicht Inf.
= C 102 sup. above (p. 41) (*Census*: 135, nr [0667]).

(f. 128) *Ars medica* (Expl. διὰ βάθους δεόμενα).
(f. 6) *De remediis parabilibus libri III* (Frgm. Περὶ ῥεουσῶν τριχῶν = K. XIV 393; liber II 2).

Mailand, Bibl. Ambrosiana, D 293 Inf.; s. XV ex.

Synopsis librorum suorum sedecim de pulsibus.

Mailand, Bibl. Ambrosiana, D 518 Inf.; s. XV ex.

Synopsis librorum suorum sedecim de pulsibus (Expl. κατὰ λόγον ὁ σφυγμὸς φαίνεται).

Mailand, Bibliotheca Trivulziana
Now Milano, Archivio Storico Civico e Biblioteca Trivulziana

Mailand, Bibl. Trivulziana, 685, s. XIV, XV (XIV).
Milano, Archivio Storico Civico e Biblioteca Trivulziana, 685.

(f. 1) *De temperamentis* (Init. mutil. inc. νοη]θῆναι = K. I 552, 4).
(f. 29) *De facultatibus naturalibus.*
(f. 75–81) *De optima corporis nostri constitutione.*
(f. 81) *De bono habitu.*
(f. 77–83) *De inaequali intemperie.*

(f. 83–86) *Distinctio.*
(f. 86–119) *Ad Glauconem de medendi methodo libri II.*
(f. 120) *In Hippocratis librum de acutorum victu commentarii IV.*
(f. 120ᵛ–122) *Sermo aversus empiricos medicos* (Frgm. Inc. ... τὸν ϛ' ἔτι θεάσασθαι περιμενεῖς. Expl. ἢ οὐκ ἂν αὐτοσχεδίως ...).
(f. 122ᵛ–193) *In Hippocratis librum de acutorum victu commentarii IV.*
(f. 193–230) *In Hippocratis praedictionum librum primum commentarii III* (Libri I et II; lib. II inc. ἂν ᾖ κατὰ μὲν τὴν χρόαν, ὕπωχρον μετρίως = K. XVI 588, 14; expl. ἢ σπόνδυλος ἐγκάθηται, τουτέοισιν = K. 678).

Messina, Universität
Now at the Biblioteca Regionale Universitaria Giacomo Longo di Messina

Messina, Universität, 84; s. –.
Now Biblioteca Regioniale Universitaria Giacomo Longo di Messina, S. Salvatore, 84.

Excerpta varia (Cf. Rühl Philol. N. F. I 577–588).

Messina, Universität, 111; s. XII.
Now Biblioteca Regioniale Universitaria Giacomo Longo di Messina, F 4/4B (*Census*: 138, nr [0683]).

Methodi medendi libri XIV (Lib. I).

Modena, Bibl. Estense
Now Modena, Biblioteca Estense Universitaria

Modena, Bibl. Estense, 61 (III B 9); s. XV.
Now α.U.9.4 (*Census*: 141, nr [0689]).

(f. 17ᵛ) *Praesagitio omnino vera expertaque* (Inc. ἔτι τὸν θέλοντα).
(f. 17ᵛ) *Lexicon botanicum* (Inc. *und* Expl. *wie im* Berolin. [Phill. 1570] [above p. 11]).
(f. 31) **Hippokrates**, **Galenos**, **Theophilus**, *Excerpta varia*.

Modena, Bibl. Estense, 78 (II C 11); s. XV.
Now α.W.2.9 (*Census*: 141, nr [0690]).

De simplicium medicamentorum temperamentis et facultatibus libri XI.

Modena, Bibl. Estense, 97 (III C 18); s. XVI.
Now α.U.9.23 (*Census*: 141, nr [0692]).

Ars medica.

Modena, Bibl. Estense, 107 (II D 8); s. X.
Now α.P.5.18 (*Census*: 141, nr [0693]).

De simplicium medicamentorum temperamentis et facultatibus libri XI.

Modena, Bibl. Estense, 109 (II D 10); s. XIV–XV.
Now α.P.5.20 (*Census*: 141, nr [0694]).

Ad Glauconem de medendi methodo libri II (Libri II. Expl. φαρμάκων ἐπιτιθέναι τι τῶν πρὸς τὰ ...).
(f. 63^{v}) *De sectis ad eos qui introducuntur.*
(f. 69) *De optima corporis nostri constitutione.*
(f. 71^{v}) *De bono habitu.*
(f. 73^{v}) *De inaequali intemperie.*

Modena, Bibl. Estense, 115 (II D 16); s. XV.
Now α.P.5.17 (*Census*: 141, nr [0695]).

(f. 9) *De urinis.*

Modena, Bibl. Estense, 151 (II E 18); s. XV.
Now α.V.7.18 (*Census*: 141, nr [0698]).

(f. 1) *Excerpta varia.*

Modena, Bibl. Estense, 175 (II F 10); s. XV.
Now α.V.7.4 (*Census*: 142, nr [0700]).

De facultatibus naturalibus.

Modena, Bibl. Estense, 210 (III G 6); s. XVI.
Now α.V.6.12 (*Census*: 142, nr [0702]).

(f. 387) *Definitiones medicae.*

Modena, Bibl. Estense, 211 (III G 7); s. XV.
Now α.G.3.11 (*Census*: 142, nr [0703]).

In Hippocratis epidemiarum libros commentarii (in Hipp. de morb. popul. Lib. I et III).

Modena, Bibl. Estense, 213; s. XV.
= α.G.3.12 (*Census*: 142, nr [0704]).
Same as **213 (III G 9)** below.

(f. 161ᵛ) *De atra bile.*

Modena, Bibl. Estense, 213 (III G 9); s. XV.
Now α.G.3.12 (*Census*: 142, nr [0705]).
See also **213** above.

(f. 3) *De locis affectis libri VI* (Expl. φαίνεσθαι τῶν καταμηνίων ἐπεχομένων).
(f. 143) *De purgantium medicamentorum facultatibus* (Expl. καὶ τοὺς καθ' ἕκαστον αὐτῶν τρόπους τῆς ἰάσευς).
(f. 154) *De dignotione ex insomniis.*
(f. 155) *Quomodo morbum simulantes sint deprehendi.*
(f. 157) *Quos, quibus catharticis medicamentis et quando purgare opporteat.*
(f. 175) *De plenitudine.*
(f. 198ᵛ) *Introductio sive medicus* (Ab initio usque ad cap. περὶ ἐμβροχῶν).

Modena, Bibl. Estense, 216 (II H 1); s. XVI.
Now α.O.4.9 (*Census*: 142, nr [0706]).

(f. 25) *De simplicium medicamentorum temperamentis et facultatibus libri XI* (Frgm. l. VI οὕτως οὖν τὸ ἀφέψημα .... ἀδήκτως ξηραίνει).
(f. 36ᵛ) *Remedia* (Frgm. ex l. de simplicibus, calefaciunt et refrigerant. Inc. Ὅσα ἐστὶ μέσα τῶν θερμαινόντων ... χρησιμώτατόν ἐστι ...).

Modena, Bibl. Estense, 217 (II H 2); s. XIV.
Now α.O.4.7 (*Census*: 142, nr [0707]).

(f. 34) *Introductio sive medicus* (Usque ad ὡς δὲ ἐκ τῶν δευτέρων, καὶ = K. XIV 696, 6).
(f. 42) *De alimentorum facultatibus libri III* (A lib. I 2 = K. VI 483, 13 usque ad cap. περὶ καθαρτηρίων).

Modena, Bibl. Estense, 218 (II H 3); s. XVI.
Now α.O.4.6 (*Census*: 142, nr [0708]).

(f. 2) *De crisibus libri III.*
(f. 102) *De morborum temporibus.*

Modena, Bibl. Estense, 219 (II H 4); s. XVI.
Now α.O.4.11 (*Census*: 142, nr [0709]).

De usu partium corporis humani libri XVII (*Am Schlusse dasselbe Epigr. wie im* [Lond.] Addit. Brit. Mus. 11, 888 [above p. 36]).

Modena, Bibl. Estense, 226 (II H 11); s. XVI.
Now α.O.4.12 (*Census*: 142, nr [0711]).

(f. 1) *De pulsuum differentiis libri IV.*
(f. 86) *De dignoscendis pulsibus libri IV.*
(f. 144) *De causis pulsuum libri IV.*
(f. 204) *De praesagitione ex pulsibus libri IV.*
(f. 271) *De anatomia, De anatomicis administrationibus libri IX* (Frgm. »De anat. intenar. et extern. partium«).

Modena, Bibl. Estense, 237 (III G 18); s. XVI.
Now α.W.3.12 (*Census*: 143, nr [0714]).

(f. 3) *In Hippocratis praedictionum librum primum commentarii III.*
(f. 93) *In Hippocratis prognosticum commentarii III.*
(f. 181) *De difficultate respirationis libri III.*
(f. 247v) *De causis respirationis.*
(f. 249) *De motu musculorum libri II.*
(f. 273) *De differentiis morborum.*
(f. 273) *De morborum causis.*
(f. 298v) *De symptomatum differentiis.*
(f. 368) *De differentiis febrium libri II* (Quaedam de febribus. Inc. ἔοικεν ὁ ἑκτικὸς πυρετός).
(f. 368) *De febribus* (Inc. Ἔοικεν ὁ ἑκτικὸς πυρετός. Expl. ὁμοίαν ποιησάμενοι τοῖς ἐφημέροις. *Ob von* Galen?).

Modena, Bibl. Estense, 240 (III F 17); s. XV–XVI.
Now α.J.6.28 (*Census*: 142, nr [0715]).

(f. 8) *Galeni in Hippocratis de natura hominis lib. commentarii II* (Expl. τὰ περὶ τὴν γῆν · οὐ μὴν κεκραμένον γε = K. XV 50, 3; Expl.: κεκραμένων [sic recte] γε.).

Moskau, Synodialbibl.
Now Государственный Исторический Музей (ГИМ), Синодальная Библиотека Московского Патриархата (Gosudarstvennyi Istoricheskii Muzei [GIM], Sinodal'naya Biblioteka Moskovskogo Patriarchata [State Historical Museum [GIM], Synodial Library of Moscow Patriarchate])

[Moskau, Synodialbibl., ?].
Now Jena, Thüringer Universitäts- und Landesbibliothek, Ms. G.B. f. 31 (*Census*: 145, nr [0719]).

Linguarum sive dictionum exoletarum Hippocratis explicatio.

[Moskau, Synodialbibl., Mosquenses complures].
= ? Sinod. 51, Sinod. 283 or Sinod. 507 (*Census*: 145, [0720]).

Opera varia.

Moskau, Synodialbibl., 51; s. XV.
Same as **52 (*so !*) = 464** below, and **464** (p. 50) and, possibly, one of the **Mosquenses complures** above.
= Sinod. 51 (*Census*: 156, nr [0722]).

De sectis ad eos qui introducuntur.

Moskau, Synodialbibl., 52 (*so!*) = 464.
Same as **51** above and **464** (p. 50), and possibly one of the **Mosquenses complures** above.
= Sinod. 51 (*Census*: 156, nr [0723]).

De sectis ad eos qui introducuntur.

Moskau, Synodialbibl., 260; a. 1630.
Now Sinod. 292 (*Census*: 146, nr [0724]).

(f. 202) *Quod animi mores corporis temperamenta sequantur.*

Moskau, Synodialbibl., 283 (= 466); s. XV.
Now Sinod. 283 (*Census*: 146, nr [0725]).
See also **466** below (p. 50).

De sectis ad eos qui introducuntur.

Moskau, Synodialbibl., 292; s. XVII.
Mosquens. 292 identisch mit Mosq. 260.
Same as **260** above.
= Sinod. 292 (*Census*: 146, nr [0726]).

Quod animi mores corporis temperamenta sequantur.

Moskau, Synodialbibl., 395; s. XVI–XVII.
Now Sinod. 303 (*Census*: 146, nr [0727]).

(f. 2^v) *De dignotione ex insomniis.*

Moskau, Synodialbibl., 464; s. XV.
Same as **51** and **52 (so !) = 464**, and possibly also, one of the **Mosquenses complures** above (all p. 49).
= Sinod. 51 (*Census*: 147, nr [0731]).

(f. 2) *De sectis ad eos qui introducuntur.*
(f. 8) *De pulsuum differentiis libri IV.*
(f. 42) *De dignoscendis pulsibus libri IV.*
(f. 67) *De causis pulsuum libri IV.*
(f. 93) *De praesagitione ex pulsibus libri IV.*
(f. 127) *Methodi medendi libri XIV.*
(f. 301^v) *Ad Glauconem de medendi methodo libri II.*
(f. 328^v) *Definitiones medicae.*

Moskau, Synodialbibl., 465; s. XV.
Now Sinod. 282 (*Census*: 147, nr [0732]).

(f. 1) *De optima corporis nostri constitutione.*
(f. 3^v) *De bono habitu.*
(f. 33) *In Hippocratis librum de acutorum victu commentarii IV* (Libri I et III).

Moskau, Synodialbibl., 466; s. XVI.
Same as **283** above (p. 49) and, possibly also, one of the **Mosquenses complures** above (p. 49).
= Sinod. 283 (*Census*: 147, nr [0733]).

(f. 1) *De sectis ad eos qui introducuntur.*
(f. 1) *De pulsibus ad tirones.*
(f. 25) *Ad Glauconem de medendi methodo libri II.*
(f. 61–63) *In Hippocratis de humoribus librum commentarii III* (Auctoris nomen deest et discrepat initium; Inc. Χυμοὶ καθ' Ἱππ. εἰσὶ ...; in fine mutil.).

(f. 78) *Puero epileptico consilium.*
(f. 84) *De optima corporis nostri constitutione.*
(f. 87) *De bono habitu.*
(f. 90) *In Hippocratis librum de fracturis commentarii III* (discrepat init.).
(f. 143) *De semine libri II.*
(f. 176v) *De elementis secundum Hippocratem.*
(f. 183v) *De temperamentis.*
(f. 219v) *De facultatibus naturalibus.*
(f. 251) *Ars medica.*
(f. 265) *Methodi medendi libri XIV.*
(f. 460) *De symptomatum differentiis.*

Moskau, Synodialbibl., 467; s. XVI.
Possibly same as one of the **Mosquenses complures** above (p. 49).
= Sinod. 507 (*Census*: 147, nr [0734]).

(f. 1) *De placitis Hippocratis et Platonis libri IX* (Libri II–IX).
(f. 96) *De atra bile.*
(f. 102v) *De parvae pilae exercitatione.*

Moskau, Synodialbibl., 468; s. XVI, XVII.
Now Sinod. 508 (*Census*: 147, nr [0735]).

(f. 1) *De remediis parabilibus libri III.*

München, Hof- und Staatsbibliothek
Now München, Bayerische Staatsbibliothek

[München, Hof- und Staatsbibliothek].
= ? *graecus* 551 below (p. 54) (*Census*: 151, nr [0741]).

Excerpta varia (Compendium ex. Gal.).

München, Hof- und Staatsbibliothek, graec. 39; s. XVI.

De morbis Excerpta (»fort. Galeni«; *ist zu streichen*).
(f. 80) *De hominis natura* (Frgm. fort. Galeni. Inc. Θαυμαστὸν γὰρ οὕτως ἀληθῶς τὸ ἀνθρώπινον σύγκραμα. *Ohne Überschrift*).
(f. 81) *De venae sectione* (Inc. Ὅτι τοῖς τὰ συνήθη πράττουσι. *Vgl.* Orib. Coll. med. VII 2).

(f. 86) *De alimentorum facultatibus libri III* (Frgm. Γαλ. προοίμιον περὶ τροφῶν δυνάμεως κατὰ στοιχεῖον. Inc. Πολλῶν καὶ λογίων, ὦ μέγιστε βασιλεῦ. Expl. *des 1. Stücks* f. 121ᵛ περὶ ὠτίδων κτέ. ἐκ τοῦ περὶ ἐκείνου λόγου διαγνωσθήσεται.

(f. 121ᵛ) *De alimentorum facultatibus libri III* (Frgm. Inscr. Σύνοψις τοῦ περὶ τροφῶν Γαλινοῦ. ὅτι τροφιμώτεροι οἶπε [sic] · περὶ πυρῶν ἤτοι ἄρτων. Inc. Ἠπιλημένοι [sic] καὶ τῷ οἴκῳ βαρύτεροι. Expl. f. 126ᵛ περὶ σκορόδων καὶ κρομύων καὶ πράσων κτέ. τοῖς γὰρ φλεγματώδεσι καὶ παχεῖς ἔχουσι χυμοὺς συμφέρει.

(f. 126ᵛ) *De alimentorum facultatibus libri III* (Frgm. Inscr. Ἐκ τοῦ τρίτου λόγου τοῦ περὶ τροφῶν. Inc. Περὶ τῆς ἀπὸ τῶν πεζῶν ζῴων τροφῆς κτέ. Αἱ σάρκες τῶν ζῴων αἵματος γεννητικαί. Expl. f. 130ᵛ εἰς δὲ οὔρησιν χείρους τῶν λευκῶν).

München, Hof- und Staatsbibliothek, graec. 71; a. 1531.

(f. 1) *Linguarum sive dictionum exoletarum Hippocratis explicatio* (Sine auctoris nomine. Inscr. Κατὰ στοιχεῖον Ἱπποκράτους λεξικόν. Inc. Ἀγκρομήλη, ἄγκιστρον. Expl. f. 8ᵛ ὅτι καὶ ὥρα ἡ φροντὶς ... ἐνιαυτοῦ).

München, Hof- und Staatsbibliothek, graec. 105; s. XVI.

(f. 218ᵛ) *Prognostica de decubitu ex mathematica scientia* (fine mutil. K. XIX 529–545; Expl. mut. ἐὰν δὲ ἀγαθοποιὸς τὴν σελήνην θεωρήσῃ = K. XIX 545, 7).

München, Hof- und Staatsbibliothek, graec. 109; s. XVI.

(f. 1) *Definitiones medicae* (Inc. Τὴν τῶν ὅρων πραγματείαν κτέ).

(f. 22) *Introductio sive medicus* (Cap. V et X desunt. *Es fehlen* Kap. V *und* XI, *nicht* X. Lücken gelassen z. B. in Kap. XII, im Abschnitt περὶ ἰσχουρίας und öfter).

(f. 50–61) *Quod animi mores corporis temperamenta sequantur* (fine mutil. [*Ist vollständig*]).

München, Hof- und Staatsbibliothek, graec. 231; s. XVI.

In Hippocratis epidemiarum libros commentarii I–III (in Libr. I et II; Inc. mut. μόνον προγνώσεται τὰς γινομένας νόσους = K. XVII A 5, 13. Expl. mut. τῶν ἔνδον τοῦ περιτοναίου μορίων, *also wie im* [Venet.] Marc. App. cl. V 15 [below p. 111], = K. XVII A 791, 19. *Der Codex enthält f.* 1–106ᵛ Comm. I–III in Epid. A', f. 106ᵛ–228ᵛ Comm. I–III in Epid. Γ').

München, Hof- und Staatsbibliothek, graec. 236; s. XV.

(f. 1) *Ad Glauconem de medendi methodo libri II.*

München, Hof- und Staatsbibliothek, graec. 276; s. XII.

(f. 5) **Hippokrates**, *Prognostica* (Προγνωστικὸν ἀῤῥώστων συγγραφὲν Ἱππ. καὶ Γαλ. καὶ Πλάτωνος καὶ σοφ. ἰατρῶν).

München, Hof- und Staatsbibliothek, graec. 278; s. XII.
ist zu streichen.

Prognostica (*Wie im* Monac. 276) (above).

München, Hof- und Staatsbibliothek, graec. 469; s. XIII, XV.
s. XIV (?).
f. 1–50: *nach alter Zählung* φυλλ. ιη'–ϙγ' *am rechten Rande (also vorher die ersten 17 Blätter verloren*); f. 1–50ᵛ: *nach neuerer Zählung am untern Rande, die öfter mehrere Blätter überspringt*; f. 51–55: *nach alter Zählung am rechten Rande* φυλλ. ϙδ'–ϙγ', *nach neuerer am unteren Rande f. 51–55ᵛ*; f. 55ᵛ: φυλλ. ϙη' *nach alter Zählung am rechten Rande.*

(f. 1–50) *In Hippocratis librum de acutorum victu commentarii IV.*
(f. 51–55) *Definitiones medicae* (Ἐρωτήματα ἰατρικῆς τέχνης = K. XIX 350–377; Inscr. f. 51 mg. dextr. Γαληνοῦ βιβλίον Α' · τὰ ἐρωτήματα τῆς ἰατρικῆς τέχνης. Inc. Τί ἐστι τέχνη; τέχνη ἐστὶ σύστημα ἐγκαταλήψεως ἐγγεγυμνασμένη = K. XIX 350, 7. Expl. ποιεῖται τὴν κίνησιν ἔν τε κύκλῳ καὶ ἐπ' εὐθείας = K. XIX 377, 6. *Vielfach von Kühns Text im einzelnen abweichend*).
(f. 55ᵛ) *De temporibus etesiarum et quomodo iis utendum sit* (Inc. Ἀπὸ πλειάδων δύσεως ἕως τροπῶν χειμερινῶν. Expl. ζήσεις ἄνοσος τὸν ὑπόλοιπον τῆς ζωῆς σου χρόνον).
(p. 56–131) *De simplicium medicamentorum temperamentis et facultatibus libri XI* (Libri VIII et IX. *Andre Hand als vorher die von* Galenus εἰς Ἱπποκρ. π. διαίτης ὀξ. *und* π. τῶν ἐτησίων καιρῶν. – Inc. mut. τρύχνου τῆς ῥίζης ὁ φλοιός = K. XII 145, 18. Also Buch VIII Ende bis Buch XI Schluß des Werkes).
(p. 132–137) *Quos, quibus catharticis medicamentis et quando purgare opporteat.*

München, Hof- und Staatsbibliothek, graec. 525; ante a. 1336.

(f. 160) *De anni temporibus* (Γαλ. ἡ τῆς τῶν ὡρῶν τάξις ... τοῦ ἔαρος).

München, Hof- und Staatsbibliothek, graec. 551; s. XV.
See also **[Hof- und Staatsbibliothek]** above (p. 51).

(f. 334) *Iatrosophia*.
(f. 353v–359v) *De podagra* (Inscr. Ἑρμηνεία περὶ τῆς ποδάγρας τοῦ σοφωτάτου Γαλ. Expl. μετὰ τοῦ p. 867 Bern).

München, Hof- und Staatsbibliothek, lat. 807; s. XV.
= Clm 807 (*Census*: 157, nr [0775]).

(f. 72) *Excerpta varia*.

Neapel, Biblioteca Borbonica
Now Napoli, Biblioteca Nazionale Vittorio Emanuele III

Neapel, Biblioteca Borbonica, III D 15; s. XIV.
See also **229 (III D 15)** below.

(f. 175) *De placitis Hippocratis et Platonis libri IX* (Frgm.).
(f. 177v–178) *De constitutione artis medicae ad Patrophilum liber*.
(f. 178v–184v) *Excerpta varia*.

Neapel, Biblioteca Borbonica, 229 (III D 15); s. XIV.
Now III D 15 above (*Census*: 162, nr [0784]).

(f. 174v) *De elementis secundum Hippocratem* (Προλεγόμενα εἰς τὸ τοῦ Γαλ. περὶ στοιχείων. Inc. Ἐπειδὴ τὰ ἀνθρώπινα σώματα).
(f. 175) *De placitis Hippocratis et Platonis libri IX*.
(f. 177v–178) *De constitutione artis medicae ad Patrophilum liber*.
(f. 178v–184v) *Excerpta varia*.
(f. 184v–193v) *De ossibus ad tirones* (mit Scholien).

Neapel, Biblioteca Borbonica, 304 D III 20; s. XIV.
Now III D 20 (*Census*: 163, nr [0785]).

De simplicium medicamentorum temperamentis et facultatibus libri XI (Frgm. Xenocratis ex libro XI).

Neapel, Bibliotheca dei Gerolamini
Now Napoli, Biblioteca statale oratoriana del Monumento nazionale dei Girolamini

Neapel, Bibl. dei Gerolamini, XXII.1; s. XIV, XV.
Now Biblioteca statale oratoriana del Monumento nazionale dei Girolamini, Pil. XXII. nr I (*Census*: 163, nr [0789]).
See also **Bibl. Oratoriana, 152** below.

(f. 167ᵛ–170) *De urinis* (Inc. *wie im* Scorial. Φ. III. 12 [above p. 19]. Expl. πολυειδῆ καὶ ἄπεπτα).
(f. 172 sq.) *De temperamentis* (Frgm. Inc. Τῶν κράσεων δύο εἰσὶ διαφοραί. Expl. τὸ γεῶδες τοῦ σπέρματος).

Neapel, Bibliotheca Oratoriana

Neapel, Bibl. Oratoriana, 152; s. XIV, XIV–XV.
Same as **Bibl. dei Gerolamini, XXII. nr 1** above (*Census*: 164, nr [0793]).
Now Biblioteca statale oratoriana del Monumento nazionale dei Girolamini, Pil. XXII. nr I.

De pulsibus.
De venae sectione.
Remedia (Quaenam medicamenta quibus infirmatatibus prosint).

Oxford, Bibl. Aedis Christi
Now Oxford, Christ Church Library

Oxford, Bibl. Aedis Christi, 34; s. XI.

(f. 131) *Excerpta varia.*

Oxford, Bibl. Bodleiana

Oxford, Bibl. Bodleiana, Baroccian. 88; s. XV–XVI, XV (XVI), XVI.
See also **[88]** below.

(f. 47) **Hippokrates**, **Paulus Italus**, **Galenos**, **Athenaeus** *Prognostica/Excerpta* (Ἱπποκρ. διδασκάλου καὶ Γαλ. σοφοῦ καὶ Παύλου Ἰτάλου καὶ Ἀθηναίου ῥήτορος καὶ Ἰωάννου Τζέτζου διάγνωσις περὶ ἰαλίων [l. ὑαλίων] ἀρρώστων καὶ τελευτῆς ἀνθρώπων. Inc. Τὸ α΄. ἄσπρον. Expl. σημαίνει καὶ θάνατον).

(f. 47 b) **Hippokrates**, **Galenos** *De urinis* (Σύνοψις ἀκριβὴς περὶ οὔρων Ἱππ. καὶ Γαλ. Inc. Ἐὰν ἔστι κλόκιον ἀνθρώπου. Expl. καὶ οὐ σύντομον θάνατον).

(f. 48 b) *De vita et morte* (Expl. ἢ καὶ τοῦ θανάτου).

(f. 48 b) *De pulsibus* (Γνωρίσματα σφυγμῶν περὶ τε ζωῆς καὶ θανάτου ἀνθρώπων. Inc. Κράτει σφυγμός. Expl. ἢ καὶ τοῦ θανάτου).

[Oxford, Bibl. Bodleiana, Baroccian. 88; s. XV (XVI)].
Same as **88** above.
= MS. *Baroccianus* 88 (*Census*: 172, nr [0818]).

De morbis Excerpta (Ex Gal. et aliis de morbis et medicamentis variis. *Vgl. unter* π. οὔρων und π. σφυγμῶν).

Oxford, Bibl. Bodleiana, Baroccian. 131; s. XIV, XIV in.

(f. 341) *De morbis Excerpta* (Προθεωρία τῆς περὶ αἰτίας περὶ διαφορᾶς νοσημάτων. Inc. Ἀρχὴ οὖν καὶ κρηπίς. Expl. ὑποκειμένου χειρήσομεν).

(f. 341) *De morborum causis* (Frgm. Προθεωρία Γαλ. τῆς περὶ αἰτίας διαφόρων νοσημάτων · ἀρχὴ οὖν καὶ κρηπὶς πάσης τῆς ἰατρικῆς τέχνης. Inc. Ὑπὲρ αἰτίας θεωρία. Expl. ὑποκειμένου χρήσομεν–).

(f. 343) *De historia philosopha.*

(f. 447 b) *Quod animi mores corporis temperamenta sequantur* (Frgm. Expl. μὴ ποιήσῃς τόδε).

(f. 477^{v}) *De dignoscendis pulsibus libri IV* (Διάγνωσις ἀκριβὴς τῶν σφυγμῶν. Expl. Ἱπποκράτους καὶ Γαληνοῦ τῶν ἐπιστήμων [sic] ἰατρῶν).

Oxford, Bibl. Bodleiana, Baroccian. 150; s. XV, XV in.

(f. 6) *Remedia* (Σκευασία τῆς πικρᾶς; *vgl. den* Lond. [Brit. Mus.] Addit. 10, 058. f. 65 [above p. 36]).

Oxford, Bibl. Bodleiana, Baroccian. 204; s. XV in., XV.

(f. 1) *Linguarum sive dictionum exoletarum Hippocratis explicatio* (»Consentit plerumque, sed paulo contractius cum Galeni lexico«).

(f. 2^{v}) *De anatomicis administrationibus libri IX* (Frgm. Inc. Ἐν πρώτῳ ἑκάστῳ = l. VI c. 1 = K. II 537, 2).

Oxford, Bibl. Bodleiana, Baroccian. 220; s. XIII.

(f. 181) *De difficultate respirationis libri III* (Libri II et III).

Oxford, Bibl. Bodleiana, Baroccian. 224; s. XV in., XV.
See also (possibly) 264 below.

(f. 1) *De venae sectione* (*Wie im* Monacens. [39] [above p. 51]. Expl. ἀλλὰ τηρεῖν καὶ αὖθις ἐπαφαιρεῖν).

Oxford, Bibl. Bodleiana, Baroccian. 264; s. XV in.
Possibly same as MS. *Baroccianus* 224 above (*Census*: 174, nr [0829]).

(f. 51 b) *De alimentorum facultatibus libri III* (Frgm. Ἐκ τοῦ γ' λόγου τοῦ περὶ τροφῶν).
(f. 54 b) *De alimentorum facultatibus libri III* (Frgm. Exc. e l. III capp. 27–30. 33. 34. 36. 37. 40–44. 52. 62. 68–71).

Oxford, Bibl. Bodleiana, Canonician. 1; s. XVI.

(f. 98) *De podagra* (Ἑρμηνεία περὶ τῆς ποδαλγίας τοῦ σοφωτάτ. Γαλ. προοίμιον. Inc. Ἐπεὶ ὥρισεν. Expl. παραδηλώσω περὶ τῆς ποδαλγικῆς νόσου).
(f. 128 b) *De dolore capitis* (Γαλ. θεραπεία εἰς κεφαλαλγίαν).

Oxford, Bibl. Bodleiana, Canonician. 44; s. XV ex.

(f. 1) *De locis affectis libri VI* (Libri VI; l. III des. τινες = K. VIII 214, 4; l. IV inc. λογικὰς διαγνώσεις = K. VIII 271, 1).
(f. 251) *De difficultate respirationis libri III* (Libri III; l. II des. δύσπνοια = K. VII 887, 6; l. III Inc. καὶ τὰ λοιπά = K. VII 890, 10).

Oxford, Bibl. Bodleiana, Clarkian. 16 (18378); s. XIV.
= MS. E. D. Clarke 16 (*Census*: 175, nr [0835]).

(f. 74 b) *De pulsibus ad Antonium* (Expl. καὶ μάλιστα ἐπὶ τῶν ἀκμαζόντων = K. XIX 641, 3).
(f. 95) *Remedia* (Περὶ ἐβένου. Inc. Ἔβενος τῶν εἰς χυλὸν ἀναλυομένων ἐστὶ ξύλων. Expl. καὶ ῥεύματα καὶ φλυκταίνας ἁρμόττουσιν).

Oxford, Bibl. Bodleiana, Is. Casauboni Advers. 4.
Now MS. Casaubon 4 (*Census*: 175, nr [0837]).

(f. 2) *De propriorum animi cuiuslibet affectuum dignotione et curatione*.

Oxford, Bibl. Bodleiana, Laud. 58 (nunc 59; Bodl. 708); s. XV.
= MS. Laud Gr. 59 (*Census*: 176, nr [0840]).

(f. 374) *De urinis* (Inc. *wie im* Lond. [Brit. Mus.] Addit. 17, 900 [above p. 36]. Expl. μαρασμὸν σημαίνει).

Oxford, Bibl. Bodleiana, Laudian. C 54 (nunc 56; Bodl. 706); s. XV in.
Now MS. Laud Gr. 56 (*Census*: 177, nr [0846]).

Methodi medendi libri XIV.

Oxford, Bibl. Bodleiana, Laudian. C 55 (nunc 57; Bodl. 707); s. XV in.
Now MS. Laud Gr. 57 (*Census*: 177, nr [0847]).

(f. 1) *De pulsuum differentiis libri IV.*
(f. 75 b) *De dignoscendis pulsibus libri IV.*
(f. 128) *De causis pulsuum libri IV.*
(f. 183) *De praesagitione ex pulsibus libri IV* (L. IV lacunos. des. περὶ κρίσεων = K. IX 429, 4).

Oxford, Bibl. Bodleiana, Laudian. C 57 (nunc 58, Bodl. 709); s. XV in.
Now MS Laud Gr. 58 (*Census*: 177, nr [0848]).

De ponderibus et mensuris.
(f. 2) *De locis affectis libri VI.*
(f. 133) *De elementis secundum Hippocratem.*
(f. 155 b) *De temperamentis.*
(f. 202 b) *De inaequali intemperie.*
(f. 208) *De facultatibus naturalibus.*
(f. 262 b) *De crisibus libri III.*
(f. 319) *De diebus decretoriis libri III.*

Oxford, Bibl. Bodleiana, Miscell. 20; s. XIV.
Now MS. Auct. E. 1. 6 (*Census*: 178, nr [0851]).

(f. 375) *De semine libri II*, *De spermate* (de spermate ex Aristotele et Galeno. Inc. Καὶ τὸ γεννητικόν).

Oxford, Bibl. Bodleiana, Miscell. 130; s. XVII.
Now MS. Auct. F. inf. 2. 1 (*Census*: 178, nr [0853]).

(p. 327) *De dignotione ex insomniis.*

Oxford, Bibl. Bodleiana, Miscell. 132; s. XVI.
Now MS. Marshall 72 (*Census*: 178, nr [0854]).

(f. 93 b) *De probis pravisque alimentorum sucis.*

Oxford, Bibl. Bodleiana, d'Orvillian. X 1. 1. 3; s. XV ex.
Now MS. D'Orville 3 (*Census*: 179, nr [0865]).
See **[Amsterdam, Universitäts-Bibliothek, Amstelodam.** ?] above (p. 5).

(f. 144) *Linguarum sive dictionum exoletarum Hippocratis explicatio.*
(f. 191) *Definitiones medicae.*
(f. 214) *Introductio sive medicus* (Capitum divisio ab usitata discrepat).

Oxford, Bibl. Bodleiana, Roe 15 (Bodl. 261); s. XV, XV ex.
= MS. Roe 15 (*Census*: 180, nr [0872]).
See also **15 (Bodl. 260 [261 *bei* Ackermann])** below.

(f. 102^{v}) *De excrementis.*

Oxford, Bibl. Bodleiana, Roe 15 (Bodl. 260 [261 *bei* Ackermann]); s. XV ex.
Same as **Roe 15 (Bodl. 261)** above.
= MS. Roe 15 (*Census*: 180, nr [0873]).

(f. 89 b) *De urinis* (Inc. *und* Expl. *wie im* Laudian. [58]) (above p. 58).

Padua, Bibl. Joann. Rhodii

Padua, Bibl. Joann. Rhodii.
Verbleib unbekannt.
Now København, Det Kongelige Bibliotek, e don. var., 42, 4° (*Census*: 190, nr [0890]) (above p. 30).

Ars medica.

Padua, Bibl. Joann. Rhodii.
Verbleib unbekannt.
Now København, Det Kongelige Bibliotek, e don. var. 29, 2° (*Census*: 191, nr [0894]).

Ad Glauconem de medendi methodo libri II.

Palermo, Biblioteca nazionale
Now Palermo, Biblioteca centrale della Regione siciliana
«Alberto Bombace»

Palermo, Biblioteca nazionale, XIII C 3; s. –, XVI.

(f. 1–44^v) **Hippokrates**, *Jatrosophium* (Ἰατροσόφ. Ἱππ. καὶ Γαλ. καὶ ἑτέρων φιλοσόφων καὶ ἰατρῶν. Inc. Περὶ ἤθους ἰατρῶν. Ποδαπὸν δεῖ εἶναι τὸν ἰητρόν. Expl. ἐν οὔρῳ, ἐν πτύσμασιν, ἐν ἱδρῶτι).

(f. 84^v–85) *De urinis* (Inc. *und* Expl. *wie im* [Oxon., Bodl.] Laudian. [58] [above p. 58]).

(f. 121–238) **Hippokrates**, **Galenos**, *Jatrosophium/Iatrosophia* (Inscr. Ἀνθολόγιον ἰατροσοφικὸν τοῦ Ἱππ. τοῦ Κῴου καὶ Γαλ. ... καὶ ἑτέρ. ἰατρῶν).

Paris, Bibl. regia

[Paris, B. R. 120 ap. Montf. II 902].
= Paris, Bibliothèque nationale de France, *Coislinianus* 163 below (p. 61) (*Census*: 195, nr [0909]).

In Hippocratis de humoribus librum commentarii III.

Paris, Bibl. Facult. Méd./ Bibl. Facult. Medic.
Now Paris, Bibliothèque Interuniversitaire de Santé – BIU Santé

Paris, Bibl. Facult. Méd., nr. ?.
Same as **Bibl. Facult Medic. 14** below.
= MS 44 (*Census*: 199, nr [0919]).

Lexicon Galeni.

Paris, Bibl. Facult. Medic. 14; s. XVII.
= MS 44 (*Census*: 199, nr [0920]).
Same as **Paris, Bibl. Facult. Méd., nr.** ? above.

(f. 73) *In Hippocratis de humoribus librum commentarii III* (e cod. Coisl. 163 descr.).

Paris, Bibl. Nationale, Coislin.
Now Paris, Bibliothèque nationale de France, Coisliniani

[Paris, Bibl. Nationale, Coislin., ap. Montf. II 447].
Same as **Coislin 334** below (p. 62) (*Census*: 200–201, nr [0926]).

De temperamentis.
De facultatibus naturalibus.

[Paris, Bibl. Nationale, Coislin., ap. Montf. II 447; s. XV].
Es ist wohl Coislin. 335.
Same as **Coislin 334** below (p. 62) (*Census*: 201, nr [0927]).

(f. 198^{v} [*gemeint*]) *De urinis* (*vgl. Unter Excerpta varia*).

[Paris, Bibl. Nationale, Coislin., ap. Montf. II 448].
Same as **Coislin 335** below (p. 62) (*Census*: 201–202, nr [0928]).

De simplicium medicamentorum temperamentis et facultatibus libri XI.

[Paris, Bibl. Nationale, Coislin., ap. Montfauc. II 448].
Same as **Coislin 335** below (p. 62) (*Census*: 202, nr [0929]).

De morbis Excerpta (Exc. ex Hipp. Gal. Meletio. *Wohl* Coislin. 335; *vgl. unter* Ἰατροσόφια).

Paris, Bibl. Nationale, Coislin., 163; a. 1560.

(f. 73) *In Hippocratis de humoribus librum commentarii III.*

Paris, Bibl. Nationale, Coislin., 228; s. XI–XIV.
Also **[Paris, B. R. 120 ap Montf. II 902]** above (p. 60).

(f. 96) *Introductio sive medicus* (pars tantum oper.).

Paris, Bibl. Nationale, Coislin., 300; a. 1318.
Now Санкт-Петербург, Российская Национальная Библиотека (РНБ), Собрание греческих рукописей, 116 (Sankt-Peterburg, Rossiiskaia natsional'naya biblioteka [RNB], Sobranie grecheskikh rukopisej, 116 – Saint Petersburg, National Library of Russia [NLR], Greek manuscripts, 116) (*Census*: 204–205, nr [0944]).

(f. 214^{v}) *Iatrosophia.*

Paris, Bibl. Nationale, Coislin., 333; s. XIV–XV.

De usu partium corporis humani libri XVII (L. I–VII).

Paris, Bibl. Nationale, Coislin., 334; s. XV.
See also **[Coislin., ap. Montf. II 447]** above (p. 61).

(f. 10) *De differentiis febrium libri II.*
(f. 10) *De febribus.*

Paris, Bibl. Nationale, Coislin., 335; s. XV.
See also **[Coislin., ap. Montf./Mountfauc. II 448]** above (p. 61).

(f. 17) *Excerpta varia.*
(f. 21) *Remedia* (*bei* Montfauc. II p. 448).
(f. 21–60) *Iatrosophia* (Jatros. Gal. Hipp. Melet. Cap. DCIV).
(f. 63) *Lexicon botanicum* (Inc. *wie im* Athous [= Βιβλ. Μον. Ἰβήρ. 4271.151] [above p. 6]).
(f. 69) *De succedaneis liber* (Inc. *wie im* Lond. [Brit. Mus.] Addit. [10, 058] [above p. 36]).
(f. 69) *Remedia* (*bei* Montfauc. II p. 448).
(f. 75) **Galenos**, **Hippokrates**, **Meletius monachus**, *Iatrosophia/Excerpta varia* (Jatros. Gal. Hipp. et Melet. Cap. DCIV).
(f. 75) *Remedia* (*bei* Montfauc. II p. 448).
(f. 198v) *De humoribus* (*bei* Montf. II 448).
(f. 198v–227) *Excerpta varia.*

Paris, Bibl. Nationale, Coislin., 336; s. XVI.

(f. 98v) *Quod animi mores corporis temperamenta sequantur.*

Paris, Bibl. Nationale, Coislin., 387; s. XI/XII.

(f. 241v) *De compositione medicamentorum secundum locos libri X* (Frgm. Εἰς τὸ τοῦ Φίλωνος βοήθημα = K. XIII 267).

Paris, Bibl. Nationale, Imprimés, Rés. Te 138.27; s. XV.

(f. 31v) *Lexicon botanicum.*

Paris, Bibl. Nationale, Parisin.
Now Paris, Bibliothèque nationale de France, *graeci*

Paris, Bibl. Nationale, Parisin. 985; s. XV, XVI.

(f. 26) *De differentiis febrium libri II.*
(f. 225) *De usu partium corporis humani libri XVII.*

Paris, Bibl. Nationale, Parisin. 1310; s. XV.

(f. 444) *De metallis* (Aristotelis et Gal. frgta. de metallis quae reperiuntur in Cypro insula. *Vgl.* Galenus XII 214. 219. 226. 239 K.).

Paris, Bibl. Nationale, Parisin. 1438; s. XVI.

(f. 275) *Introductio sive medicus.*

Paris, Bibl. Nationale, Parisin. 1630; s. XIV.

(f. 19) *De pulsibus ad Antonium* (Frgm. *Vgl.* Rhein. Mus. 47 S. 456[3]).
(f. 216) *De podagra* (Frgm. de podagra. Inc. Ἐκ τοῦ γένους. Cf. K. XIII 334).

Paris, Bibl. Nationale, Parisin. 1644; s. XV.

(f. 38) *Ars medica.*

[Paris, Bibl. Nationale, Parisin. 1819 (? = 1849 ?)].
Same as **1849** below (*Census*: 212, nr [1007]).

De anatomicis administrationibus libri IX.

Paris, Bibl. Nationale, Parisin. 1831; s. XVI.

(f. 119) *Excerpta varia* (Frgm. Inc. θυμοῦσιν οὐκέτι ὁμοίως).

Paris, Bibl. Nationale, Parisin. 1849; s. XIV.
See also **[1819 (? = 1849 ?)]** above.

(f. 9) *De anatomicis administrationibus libri IX.*
(f. 95) *De motu musculorum libri II.*
(f. 111) *In Hippocratis de articulis librum commentarii IV.*
(f. 147^{v}) *In Hippocratis librum de fracturis commentarii III.*
(f. 175^{v}) *In Hippocratis librum de officina medici commentarii III.*

Paris, Bibl. Nationale, Parisin. 1865; s. XV.

(f. 129) *Excerpta varia.*

Paris, Bibl. Nationale, Parisin. 1883; s. XIV.

(f. 29v) *De sectis ad eos qui introducuntur.*
(f. 35v) *De elementis* (Frgm. »de quattuor elementis«).
(f. 36v) *Ars medica.*
(f. 47v) *De differentiis febrium libri II.*
(f. 156v) *De alimentorum facultatibus libri III* (Libri II; Expl. L. II c. 21).
(f. 785v) *De succedaneis liber.*

Paris, Bibl. Nationale, Parisin. 1884; a. 1503.

(f. 158) *Hippocratis aphorismi et Galeni in eos commentarii VII.*

Paris, Bibl. Nationale, Parisin. 1949; s. XV.

(f. 418v) *De symptomatum causis libri III* (Frgm.).

Paris, Bibl. Nationale, Parisin. 1991; s. XV.

(f. 29) *Prognostica de decubitu ex mathematica scientia* (*Abschrift des* [Florent.] Laurent. 28, 34 [above p. 20]).
(f. 29v–42) *De chirurgorum operationibus et de decubitu infirmorum.*

Paris, Bibl. Nationale, Parisin. 2091; s. XV.

(f. 8) *De hominis natura testamentum. De victu singulis mensibus servando* (Frgm.).

[Paris, Bibl. Nationale, Parisin. 2113 (?)].
= ? **2153** below (p. 66) (*Census*: 215, nr [1035]).

Introductio sive medicus.

[Paris, Bibl. Nationale, Parisin. 2123 (?)].
= ? **2173** below (p. 71) (*Census*: 215, nr [1037]).

De compositione medicamentorum secundum locos libri X.

[Paris, Bibl. Nationale, Parisin. 2137 (?)].
= ? **2167** below (p. 69) (*Census*: 215, nr [1038]).

De causis pulsuum libri IV.

[Paris, Bibl. Nationale, Parisin. 2139 (?)].

Prognostica de decubitu ex mathematica scientia.

Paris, Bibl. Nationale, Parisin. 2140; s. XII–XIII.

(f. 1) *Linguarum sive dictionum exoletarum Hippocratis explicatio.*

Paris, Bibl. Nationale, Parisin. 2141; s. XV.

(f. 1) *Linguarum sive dictionum exoletarum Hippocratis explicatio.*

Paris, Bibl. Nationale, Parisin. 2142; s. XIII–XIV.

(f. 1) *Linguarum sive dictionum exoletarum Hippocratis explicatio.*

Paris, Bibl. Nationale, Parisin. 2143; s. XIV.

(f. 1^{v}) *Linguarum sive dictionum exoletarum Hippocratis explicatio.*

Paris, Bibl. Nationale, Parisin. 2144; s. XIV.

(f. 1) *Linguarum sive dictionum exoletarum Hippocratis explicatio.*

Paris, Bibl. Nationale, Parisin. 2145; s. XV.

(f. 1) *Linguarum sive dictionum exoletarum Hippocratis explicatio.*

Paris, Bibl. Nationale, Parisin. 2147; s. XVI.

Scholia in Galenum (»Probe bei Daremberg, Gal. in Timaeum«).

Paris, Bibl. Nationale, Parisin. 2148; s. XV.

(f. 67) *De simplicium medicamentorum temperamentis et facultatibus libri XI* (Libri II fine mutil.).
(f. 123) *De usu partium corporis humani libri XVII.*

Paris, Bibl. Nationale, Parisin. 2149; s. XVI.

(f. 159) **Oribasius**, *De ponderibus et mensuris* (De mensuris et ponderibus ex Orib. et Gal.).
(f. 201) **Galenos**, **Oribasius**, *Excerpta varia* (Orib. et Gal. capita varia de re medica).

Paris, Bibl. Nationale, Parisin. 2151; s. XVI.

(f. 97) *Lexicon botanicum* (Frgm.).

Paris, Bibl. Nationale, Parisin. 2153; XV.
Possibly also **[2113 (?)]** above (p. 64) and **[2158 (?)]** below (p. 67).

(f. 1) *Introductio sive medicus.*
(f. 81) *De dignoscendis pulsibus libri IV.*
(f. 218) *De gynaeceis i. e. de passionibus mulierum* (de morbis mulierum).

Paris, Bibl. Nationale, Parisin. 2154; s. XIV.

(f. 1) *De usu partium corporis humani libri XVII* (Libri III in. mut. – XVII. ἤ τινα τῶν = K. IV 359, 16).

Paris, Bibl. Nationale, Parisin. 2155; s. XIV.

(f. 1) *De usu partium corporis humani libri XVII* (»Superest tantum pagina una«).
(f. 2) *De compositione medicamentorum secundum locos libri X* (Libri I–IX).
(f. 292) *Excerpta varia.*
(f. 307^{v}) *De differentiis febrium libri II* (init. et fine mut.).
(f. 315^{v}) *Synopsis librorum suorum sedecim de pulsibus* (Liber de pulsibus, fine mutil.).
(f. 315^{v}–319^{v}) *De pulsibus* (Frgm.).

Paris, Bibl. Nationale, Parisin. 2156; s. XV.

(f. 1) *De differentiis febrium libri II.*
(f. 33) *Introductio sive medicus.*
(f. 47) *De morbis Excerpta* (de morborum curatione. Init. deest).
(f. 64^{v}) *De humoribus.*
(f. 176^{v}) *De simplicium medicamentorum temperamentis et facultatibus libri XI.*
(f. 358) *De compositione medicamentorum per genera libri VII* (Libri III).

[Paris, Bibl. Nationale, Parisin. 2156 (?)].
Possibly same as **2166** below (p. 69) (*Census*: 221–222, nr [1074]).

Ad Glauconem de medendi methodo libri II.

Paris, Bibl. Nationale, Parisin. 2157; s. XV.
See also (possibly) **[2175 (?)]** below (p. 71).

(f. 1) *De simplicium medicamentorum temperamentis et facultatibus libri XI.*
(f. 217) *Ad Glauconem de medendi methodo libri II.*
(f. 256) *De locis affectis Libri VI.*
(f. 369) *De differentiis morborum.*
(f. 376) *De morborum causis.*
(f. 383) *De symptomatum differentiis.*
(f. 390v) *De symptomatum causis libri III.*
(f. 425) *Methodi medendi libri XIV* (Libri III primi fine mutil.).

[Paris, Bibl. Nationale, Parisin. 2157 (?)].
Same as **2167** below (p. 69) (*Census*: 222, nr [1076]).

De differentiis febrium libri II.
De dignoscendis pulsibus libri IV.
De praesagitione ex pulsibus libri IV.
De pulsuum differentiis libri IV.

Paris, Bibl. Nationale, Parisin. 2158; s. XV.

(f. 1) *De differentiis febrium libri II.*
(f. 33) *Introductio sive medicus.*
(f. 47) *De morbis Excerpta* (*Wie im* Paris. 2156) (above p. 66).
(f. 64v) *De humoribus.*
(f. 167) *De simplicium medicamentorum temperamentis et facultatibus libri XI.*
(f. 312) *De compositione medicamentorum per genera libri VII* (Libri III).

[Paris, Bibl. Nationale, Parisin. 2158 (?)].
Possibly same as **2153** above (p. 66) (*Census*: 222, nr [1078]).

De dignoscendis pulsibus libri IV.

Paris, Bibl. Nationale, Parisin. 2159; a. 1492.

De simplicium medicamentorum temperamentis et facultatibus libri XI.

Paris, Bibl. Nationale, Parisin. 2160; a. 1473.
See also (possibly) **[2169 (?)]** below (p. 70).

(f. 1) *Methodi medendi libri XIV.*

[Paris, Bibl. Nationale, Parisin. 2160 (?)].
Possibly same as **2260** below (p. 75) (*Census*: 223, nr [1081]).

De simplicium medicamentorum temperamentis et facultatibus libri XI.

Paris, Bibl. Nationale, Parisin. 2161; s. XV.

(f. 1) *Hippocratis aphorismi et Galeni in eos commentarii VII.*
(f. 163) *De locis affectis libri VI.*
(f. 283) *De pulsuum differentiis libri IV.*
(f. 353^{v}) *De dignoscendis pulsibus libri IV.*
(f. 406) *De causis pulsuum libri IV.*
(f. 460^{v}) *De praesagitione ex pulsibus libri IV.*

Paris, Bibl. Nationale, Parisin. 2162; s. XV–XVI.
See also (possibly) **[2262 (?)]** below (p. 75).

(f. 1) *Methodi medendi libri XIV.*

Paris, Bibl. Nationale, Parisin. 2163; s. XIV.

Ars medica.

Paris, Bibl. Nationale, Parisin. 2164; s. XVI.
See also (possibly) **[2167 (?)]**, **[2169 (?)]** (p. 70), and **2664** below (p. 82).

(f. 1) *De foetuum formatione.*
(f. 14^{v}) *An animal sit quod est in utero.*
(f. 28) *De instrumento odoratus.*
(f. 35) *Quod optimus medicus sit etiam philosophus.*
(f. 37^{v}) *De parvae pilae exercitatione.*
(f. 40) *Quod qualitates incorporeae sint.*
(f. 44^{v}) *Adversus Lycum.*
(f. 56) *Thrasybulus sive utrum medicinae sit an gymnastices hygieine.*
(f. 76^{v}) *De venarum arteriarumque dissectione.*
(f. 88) *De nervorum dissectione.*
(f. 91) *De motu musculorum libri II.*
(f. 111) *De alimentorum facultatibus libri III.*
(f. 169) *De probis pravisque alimentorum sucis.*

(f. 185) *De tumoribus praeter naturam.*
(f. 191) *De theriaca ad Pisonem liber.*
(f. 213) *Remedia* (De salibus).
(f. 215) *De theriaca ad Pamphilianum.*
(f. 269) *De compositione medicamentorum secundum locos libri X* (lib. I. II).

Paris, Bibl. Nationale, Parisin. 2165; s. XVI.

(f. 1) *In Hippocratis epidemiarum libros commentarii* (in libros III).
(f. 118) *De difficultate respirationis libri III.*
(f. 164) *De plenitudine.*
(f. 177v) *De uteri dissectione.*
(f. 181v) *De urinis.*
(f. 187) *De causis respirationis.*
(f. 188) *De purgantium medicamentorum facultatibus.*
(f. 192) *De praenotione* (»praenotiones«).
(f. 195) *De dignotione ex insomniis.*
(f. 195v) *Quomodo morbum simulantes sint deprehendi.*
(f. 197) *Quos, quibus catharticis medicamentis et quando purgare opporteat.*
(f. 203) *De symptomatum differentiis.*
(f. 213) *De symptomatum causis libri III.*
(f. 258) *In Hippocratis librum de acutorum victu commentarii IV.*

Paris, Bibl. Nationale, Parisin. 2166; s. XV–XVI.
See possibly **[2156 (?)]** above (p. 67).

(f. 1) *Ad Glauconem de medendi methodo libri II* (Libri II fine mut.).
(f. 35) *De difficultate respirationis libri III* (Liber I fine mutil.).
(f. 51) *De plenitudine.*
(f. 70) *Quos, quibus catharticis medicamentis et quando purgare opporteat.*
(f. 73v) *De atra bile.*
(f. 89) *In Hippocratis praedictionum librum primum commentarii III.*

Paris, Bibl. Nationale, Parisin. 2167; s. XVI.
See also **[2137 (?)]** (possibly) (p. 65) and **[2157 (?)]** (p. 67) above.

(f. 1) *De alimentorum facultatibus libri III* (Libri II, init. et fin. mut.).
(f. 188) *De differentiis febrium libri II.*
(f. 202) *De differentiis febrium libri II* (de febrium causis).
(f. 202) *De febribus* (De febrium causis).
(f. 223) *De differentiis morborum.*
(f. 235v) *De morborum causis.*

(f. 249) *Introductio sive medicus.*
(f. 269[v]) *Definitiones medicae.*
(f. 287) *De pulsuum differentiis libri IV.*
(f. 303) *De dignoscendis pulsibus libri IV.*
(f. 343) *De causis pulsuum libri IV.*
(f. 387) *De praesagitione ex pulsibus libri IV.*

[Paris, Bibl. Nationale, Parisin. 2167 (?); s. XVI].
Possibly same as **2164** above (p. 68) (*Census*: 224, nr [1089]).

De compositione medicamentorum secundum locos libri X.

Paris, Bibl. Nationale, Parisin. 2168; s. XVI.

(f. 1) *Hippocratis aphorismi et Galeni in eos commentarii VII.*
(f. 172) *In Hippocratis praedictionum librum primum commentarii III.*
(f. 172) *In Hippocratis prognosticum commentarii III.*

Paris, Bibl. Nationale, Parisin. 2169; s. XVI.

(f. 1) *De differentiis morborum.*
(f. 11[v]) *De morborum causis.*
(f. 22) *De symptomatum differentiis.*
(f. 32[v]) *De symptomatum causis libri III.*
(f. 82[v]) *Ars medica.*
(f. 83) *Methodi medendi libri XIV* (Libri IV).

[Paris, Bibl. Nationale, Parisin. 2169 (?)].
Possibly same as **2160** (p. 68) and **2164** (p. 68) above (*Census*: 224, nr [1092]).

Introductio sive medicus.
Quod optimus medicus sit etiam philosophus.

Paris, Bibl. Nationale, Parisin. 2170; s. XVI.
See also (possibly) **[2170 (?)]** below.

(f. 1) *De simplicium medicamentorum temperamentis et facultatibus libri XI.*
(f. 248) *De periodis.*

[Paris, Bibl. Nationale, Parisin. 2170 (?)].
Same as **2270** below (p. 76) and possiby **2170** above (*Census*: 225, nr [1094]).

De totius morbi temporibus.
De typis.

Paris, Bibl. Nationale, Parisin. 2171; s. XVI.

(f. 1) *Methodi medendi libri XIV.*
(f. 209) *Introductio sive medicus.*

Paris, Bibl. Nationale, Parisin. 2172; s. XVI.

De sanitate tuenda libri VI (fine mutil.).

Paris, Bibl. Nationale, Parisin. 2173; s. XVI.
See possibly **[2123 (?)]** above (p. 64).

(f. 6) *De alimentorum facultatibus libri III.*
(f. 71) *De compositione medicamentorum secundum locos libri X.*

Paris, Bibl. Nationale, Parisin. 2174; s. XVI.

(f. 1) *In Hippocratis epidemiarum libros commentarii* (in libr. II).
(f. 106) *In Hippocratis epidemiarum libros commentarii* (in libr. III).

Paris, Bibl. Nationale, Parisin. 2175; s. XVI.

(f. 1) *Introductio sive medicus.*
(f. 50) *Definitiones medicae.*

[Paris, Bibl. Nationale, Parisin. 2175 (?)].
Possibly same as **2157** above (p. 67) (*Census*: 225, nr [1100]).

Ars medica.

Paris, Bibl. Nationale, Parisin. 2176; s. XVI.

(f. 4) *De partibus philosophiae.*

Paris, Bibl. Nationale, Parisin. 2177; s. XVI.

(f. 1) *In Hippocratis de humoribus librum commentarii III* (Frgm.).

Paris, Bibl. Nationale, Parisin. 2178; s. XIV, XV.

(f. 1) *De pulsibus* (Exc. de pulsibus).
(f. 11^{v}) *De differentiis febrium libri II* (Frgm. Exc. de febrium differentiis).
(f. 42) *De morbis Excerpta* (De morbis hominum et remediis).

Paris, Bibl. Nationale, Parisin. 2183; s. XV.

(f. 164v) *De theriaca* (Formulae theriacae).

Paris, Bibl. Nationale, Parisin. 2195; s. XIII.

(f. 467v) *De theriaca ad Pisonem liber.*

Paris, Bibl. Nationale, Parisin. 2207; a. 1299 (1294).

(f. 217) *De pulsibus ad tirones* (Frgm.).

[Paris, Bibl. Nationale, Parisin. 2208 (?)].
Possibly same as **2238** below (p. 73) (*Census*: 227, nr [1134]).

De succedaneis liber.

Paris, Bibl. Nationale, Parisin. 2210; a. 1357 (1537).

(f. –) *De septimestri partu.*
(f. 368) *Excerpta varia.*

Paris, Bibl. Nationale, Parisin. 2219; s. XV.

(f. 74) *Hippocratis aphorismi et Galeni in eos commentarii VII* (Libri II–VI, init. mutil.).
(f. 124v) *De musculorum dissectione.*
(f. 140v) *De nervorum dissectione.*

Paris, Bibl. Nationale, Parisin. 2224; s. XIV ex., XIV–XV, XV.

(f. 42) **Hippokrates**, **Galenos**, *De urinis* (ex Gal. Hipp. etc. de urinis).
(f. 44) *De excrementis.*

Paris, Bibl. Nationale, Parisin. 2228; s. XI, XII, XIV–XV.

(f. 45) *De venae sectione* (K. XIX 519–528).
(f. 48v) *De laterum morbo ad Patrophilum* (Expl. κἂν ἐγὼ μὴ λέγω).
(f. 63) **Philagrius**, **Galenos**, *Excerpta varia* (Opusculum de urinis, ex Galeno, Philagrio etc.).
(f. 66) *In Hippocratis praedictionum librum primum commentarii III.*

Paris, Bibl. Nationale, Parisin. 2229; s. XIII, XIV.

(f. 43v) *Synopsis librorum suorum sedecim de pulsibus* (Tract. de pulsibus).

(f. 43^{v}) *De pulsibus* (Frgm.).

Paris, Bibl. Nationale, Parisin. 2230; s. XIV.
See also **[2230]** below.

(f. 120) *De diaeta et morbis curandis.*

[Paris, Bibl. Nationale, Parisin. 2230; s. XIV].
Possibly same as **2230** above (*Census*: 229, nr [1157]).

De morbis Excerpta (De variis morborum generibus remediisque ad illorum curam maxime idoneis. *Es ist wohl* f. 120: De diaeta et morbis curandis *gemeint*).
Remedia (*Es ist* f. 37 Anonymi collectio medica ex variis Gal. operibus *gemeint*; *vgl.* Costomiris, Rev. des ét gr. II [1889] p. 377).

Paris, Bibl. Nationale, Parisin. 2232; s. XV.

(f. 88) *Methodi medendi libri XIV* (Liber III fine mut.).

Paris, Bibl. Nationale, Parisin. 2237; s. XIV.

(f. 165^{v}) **Oribasius**, **Galenos**, **Aëtius Amidenus**, *Excerpta varia* (Collectionis medicinalis ex Galeno Orib. Aetio libri IV–X).

Paris, Bibl. Nationale, Parisin. 2238; s. XV.
See also **[2208 (?)]** above (p. 72).

(f. 593) *De succedaneis liber.*

Nationale, Bibl. Nationale, Parisin. 2240; s. XVI.

(f. 146^{v}) *De venereis* (Frgm.).

[Paris, Bibl. Nationale, Parisin. 2245 (?)].
Same as **2247** or **2248** (p. 74) below (*Census*: 230–231, nr [1171]).

De fasciis.

Paris, Bibl. Nationale, Parisin. 2246; s. XVI.

(f. 71) *De differentiis febrium libri II.*
(f. 111) *De crisibus libri III.*
(f. 172) *De diebus decretoriis libri III.*
(f. 231) *Introductio sive medicus.*

Paris, Bibl. Nationale, Parisin. 2247; s. XVI.
See also **[2245 (?)]** above (p. 73), and **[2247 (?)]** below.

In Hippocratis de articulis librum commentarii IV.

[Paris, Bibl. Nationale, Parisin. 2247 (?)].
Same as **2247** above (*Census*: 231, nr [1175]).

De fasciis.

Paris, Bibl. Nationale, Parisin. 2248; s. XVI.
See also **[2245 (?)]** above (p. 73), possibly **2248 (?)** below.

In Hippocratis de articulis librum commentarii IV.

Paris, Bibl. Nationale, Parisin. 2248 (?); s. XVI.
Possibly same as **2248** above (*Census*: 231–232, nr [1177]).

De fasciis.

[Paris, Bibl. Nationale, Parisin. 2252 (?)].
Possibly same as **2282** below (p. 78) (*Census*: 232, nr [1183]).

Definitiones medicae.

Paris, Bibl. Nationale, Parisin. 2253; s. XI.

(f. 145) *De usu partium corporis humani libri XVII* (Libri X. XIV. XV cuius una pagina superest).

Paris, Bibl. Nationale, Parisin. 2255; s. XV.

(f. 27) *Linguarum sive dictionum exoletarum Hippocratis explicatio.*

Paris, Bibl. Nationale, Parisin. 2256; s. XIV, XV.

(f. 535v–538v) *De cruditate.*

Paris, Bibl. Nationale, Parisin. 2257; s. XVI.

(f. 120) **Hippokrates**, *Aphorismi* (Gal. in Aph. comm.; des. in aph. αἱ λεπταὶ καὶ ἀκριβέες).
(f. 129) *In Hippocratis prognosticum commentarii III.*

Paris, Bibl. Nationale, Parisin. 2260; s. XVI.
See also (possibly) **[2160 (?)]** above (p. 68) and (possibly) **[2280 (?)]** below (p. 78).

(f. 33) *De urinis.*
(f. 120[v]) *De pulsibus ad tirones.*
(f. 138) *De differentiis febrium libri II.*
(f. 196) *Remedia* (De simplicibus medicamentis).
(f. 386) *Ad Glauconem de medendi methodo libri II.*

[Paris, Bibl. Nationale, Parisin. 2262 (?)].
Possibly same as **2162** above (p. 68) (*Census*: 236, nr [1201]).

Methodi medendi libri XIV.

Paris, Bibl. Nationale, Parisin. 2265; s. XIII.

(f. 1) *Ars medica.*
(f. 76[v]) *Ad Glauconem de medendi methodo libri II.*

Paris, Bibl. Nationale, Parisin. 2266; s. XIII, XIV.

(f. 1) *In Hippocratis prognosticum commentarii III.*
(f. 93) *Hippocratis aphorismi et Galeni in eos commentarii VII.*

Paris, Bibl. Nationale, Parisin. 2267; s. XIV, XV.

De facultatibus naturalibus.
(f. 1) *De differentiis febrium libri II.*
(f. 63) *De ptisana.*
(f. 71[v]) *De temperamentis.*
(f. 255) *De elementis secundum Hippocratem.*

Paris, Bibl. Nationale, Parisin. 2268; s. XIV, XVI.

Hippocratis aphorismi et Galeni in eos commentarii VII.

Paris, Bibl. Nationale, Parisin. 2269; s. XV.

(f. 1) *Ad Glauconem de medendi methodo libri II.*
(f. 114) *Praesagitio omnino vera expertaque.*
(f. 118) *De venae sectione.*
(f. 128) *De urinis* (De praesagitione ex urinis).
(f. 145[v]) *De praenotione.*

(f. 151v) *De paroxysmorum temporibus.*
(f. 163) *De febribus* (De febri semitertiana anon.), *De differentiis febrium libri II* (Frgm. de febri semitertiana).
(f. 165v) *De uteri dissectione.*
(f. 174) *De dignotione ex insomniis.*
(f. 175v) *Quomodo morbum simulantes sint deprehendi.*
(f. 178) *De hirudinibus, revulsione, cucurbitula, incisione et scarificatione.*
(f. 180) *De tumoribus praeter naturam.*
(f. 183) *De totius morbi temporibus.*
(f. 193) *Puero epileptico consilium.*
(f. 201v) *De atra bile.*
(f. 219) *De tremore, palpitatione, convulsione et rigore.*

Paris, Bibl. Nationale, Parisin. 2270; s. XV–XVI.
See also **[2170 (?)]** above (p. 70).

(f. 1) *Introductio sive medicus.*
(f. 55) *De paroxysmorum temporibus.*
(f. 71) *De totius morbi temporibus.*
(f. 84v) *De uteri dissectione.*
(f. 94v) *Puero epileptico consilium.*
(f. 104v) *De atra bile.*
(f. 124) *De tremore, palpitatione, convulsione et rigore.*
(f. 148) *Ars medica.*
(f. 177) *De gynaeceis i. e. de passionibus mulierum.*

Paris, Bibl. Nationale, Parisin. 2271; s. XV.

(f. 1) *Ars medica.*
(f. 41) *Introductio sive medicus.*
(f. 75) *De morborum temporibus.*
(f. 95v) *Introductio sive medicus* (de oculorum affectibus = Εἰσ. cap. XVI. XVII).
(f. 107v) *De tremore, palpitatione, convulsione et rigore.*
(f. 128) *De uteri dissectione.*
(f. 135) *Puero epileptico consilium.*
(f. 142v) *De atra bile.*

Paris, Bibl. Nationale, Parisin. 2272; s. XV.

(f. 1) *De differentiis febrium libri II.*
(f. 41) *De crisibus libri III.*
(f. 101v) *De diebus decretoriis libri III.*

Paris, Bibl. Nationale, Parisin. 2273; s. XV.

(f. 3) *Ars medica.*

Paris, Bibl. Nationale, Parisin. 2274; s. XV.

Methodi medendi libri XIV.

Paris, Bibl. Nationale, Parisin. 2276; s. XVI.

(f. 1) *In Hippocratis vel Polybi opus de salubri victus ratione privatorum commentarius.*
(f. 1) *In Hippocratis librum de acutorum victu commentarii IV.*
(f. 147) *De differentiis febrium libri II.*
(f. 179ᵛ) *De dignotione ex insomniis.*
(f. 199) *De pulsibus ad tirones.*

Paris, Bibl. Nationale, Parisin. 2277; s. XV–XVI.
See (possibly) **[2278 (?)]** below.

(f. 2) *Ars medica.*
(f. 111) *De placitis Hippocratis et Platonis libri IX* (Frgm. Exc. ex libr. II–IX. Inc. *wie im* [Flor.] Laurent. 74, 12 [above p. 23]. Expl. ὡς χείροσι τοῦ λογιστικοῦ).

Paris, Bibl. Nationale, Parisin. 2278; s. XVI.

(f. 1) *De motu musculorum libri II* (Libri II in fine mut.).
(f. 1) *Hippocratis aphorismi et Galeni in eos commentarii VII* (initio et fine mutil.).

[Paris, Bibl. Nationale, Parisin. 2278 (?)].
Possibly same as **2277** above (*Census*: 240, nr [1224]).

Ars medica.
De placitis Hippocratis et Platonis libri IX (L. II–IX).

Paris, Bibl. Nationale, Parisin. 2279; s. XVI.

(f. 1) *De simplicium medicamentorum temperamentis et facultatibus libri XI* (Libri V).
(f. 155ᵛ) *De semine libri II.*

Paris, Bibl. Nationale, Parisin. 2280; s. XVI.

(f. 1) *Methodi medendi libri XIV.*
(f. 389) *Introductio sive medicus.*

[Paris, Bibl. Nationale, Parisin. 2280 (?)].
Possibly same as **2260** above (p. 75) (*Census*: 240, nr [1227]).

De simplicium medicamentorum temperamentis et facultatibus libri XI.

Paris, Bibl. Nationale, Parisin. 2281; s. XVI.

(f. 1) *De usu partium corporis humani libri XVII.*

Paris, Bibl. Nationale, Parisin. 2282; s. XVI.
See also (possibly) **[2252 (?)]** above (p. 74).

(f. 1) *Introductio sive medicus.*
(f. 53^{v}) *Definitiones medicae.*

Paris, Bibl. Nationale, Parisin. 2283; s. XVI.

De atra bile (Frgm.).
De bono habitu (Frgm.).
De crisibus libri III (Frgm.).
De diebus decretoriis libri III (Frgm.).
De differentiis febrium libri II (Frgm.).
De differentiis morborum (Frgm.).
De elementis secundum Hippocratem (Frgm.).
De inaequali intemperie (Frgm.).
De marcore (Frgm.).
De morborum causis (Frgm.).
De morborum temporibus (Frgm.).
De musculorum dissectione (Frgm.).
De optima corporis nostri constitutione (Frgm.).
De placitis Hippocratis et Platonis libri IX (Frgm.).
De praenotione (Frgm. Exc. ex »προγνωστικ. ὑπομνήματ.«).
De sanitate tuenda libri VI (Frgm.).
De sectis ad eos qui introducuntur (Frgm.).
De symptomatum causis libri III (Frgm.).
De symptomatum differentiis (Frgm.).
De temperamentis (Frgm.).
De usu partium corporis humani libri XVII (Frgm.).

De tremore, palpitatione, convulsione et rigore (Frgm.).
Methodi medendi libri XIV (Frgm. Exc. e θεραπευτικὴ μεγάλη).
Prognostica (Προγνωστ. ὑπομνήμ.).

Paris, Bibl. Nationale, Parisin. 2284; s. XVI.

De symptomatum causis libri III.

Paris, Bibl. Nationale, Parisin. 2285; s. XVI.

Ars medica.

Paris, Bibl. Nationale, Parisin. 2286; s. XIV.

(f. 89) **Archigenes**, **Asclepiades**, **Diocles**, **Timocrates**, **Galenos**, *Excerpta* (Remedia ad sedandos dentium dolores).
(f. 103) *Remedia* (Remedia varia).

Paris, Bibl. Nationale, Parisin. 2287; s. XV–XVI.

(f. 191) *Linguarum sive dictionum exoletarum Hippocratis explicatio.*

Paris, Bibl. Nationale, Parisin. 2294; s. XV.

(f. 68v) *De urinis.*
(f. 73v) *Remedia.*
(f. 101) *De succedaneis liber.*

Paris, Bibl. Nationale, Parisin. 2304; s. XV.

(f. 155v) *Ad Glauconem de medendi methodo libri II.*

[Paris, Bibl. Nationale, Parisin. 2304 (?)].
Possibly same as **2307** below (p. 80) (*Census*: 242, nr [1253]).

Ars medica.
Introductio sive medicus.

Paris, Bibl. Nationale, Parisin. 2306; s. XV.

(f. 345) *Introductio sive medicus.*
(f. 360) *Ars medica.*

Paris, Bibl. Nationale, Parisin. 2307; s. XVI.
See also (possibly) **[2304 (?)]** above (p. 79).

(f. 531^{v}) *Introductio sive medicus.*
(f. 554) *Ars medica.*

Paris, Bibl. Nationale, Parisin. 2308; s. XV.

(f. 115 [= f. 15]) *De urinis.*
(f. 160^{v}) *Ad Glauconem de medendi methodo libri II.*
(f. 249) *De insomniis.*

Paris, Bibl. Nationale, Parisin. 2309; s. XVI.

(f. 49) *De urinis.*

Paris, Bibl. Nationale, Parisin. 2312; s. XV.

(f. 422) *De succedaneis liber.*

Paris, Bibl. Nationale, Parisin. 2313; s. XIV.

(f. 1) *Remedia.*
(f. 393^{v}) *Synopsis librorum suorum sedecim de pulsibus* (Liber de pulsibus).
(f. 393^{v}–400) *De pulsibus ad Antonium.*

Paris, Bibl. Nationale, Parisin. 2316; s. XV.

(f. 191) **Mangens (?)**, **Galenos**, *De urinis*, *De urinis compendium* (Galeni et Mangentis synopsis de urinis).
(f. 215) *De differentiis morborum* (De morborum formis).
(f. 439^{v}) *De hominis natura testamentum. De victu singulis mensibus servando* (Liber de iis quae singulis mensibus servanda sunt).

Paris, Bibl. Nationale, Parisin. 2317; s. XVI.

(f. 21^{v}) *De elementis* (Frgm.), *De elementis secundum Hippocratem* (Frgm. »de quattuor elementis«).
(f. 43^{v}) *De elementis* (Frgm.), *De elementis secundum Hippocratem* (Frgm. »de elementis et humoribus«).
(f. 43^{v}) *De humoribus* (Exc. de elementis et humoribus).

Paris, Bibl. Nationale, Parisin. 2318; s. XV.
See also (possibly) **[2319 (?)]** below.

(f. 72) *De succedaneis liber.*

[Paris, Bibl. Nationale, Parisin. 2319 (?)].
Possibly same as **2318** above (*Census*: 243, nr [1266]).

De succedaneis liber.

Paris, Bibl. Nationale, Parisin. 2320; s. XVI.

(f. 1) *De demonstrationibus* (Ἱππ. καὶ Γαλ. καὶ ἑτέρων φιλοσόφων ... περὶ θεωρημάτων τε καὶ ἐπιστάσεων ἀληθοῦς ἀποδείξεως. Inc. Ὁ νόμος μὲν πάντα κρατύνει. *Vgl.* Costomiris Rev. des ét. gr. II [1889] 378–380).
(f. 9ᵛ) *De venae sectione.*
(f. 20ᵛ) *De vasis vitreis* (Μέθοδος τῶν ὑαλίων).
(f. 23) *De vita et morte* (*Wie im* [Oxford, Bodl.] Baroccian. [88]) (above p. 56).
(f. 23) *De pulsibus* (*Wie im* [Oxford, Bodl.] Baroccian. [88]).

Paris, Bibl. Nationale, Parisin. 2324; s. XVI.

(f. 1) **Galenos**, **Erasistratus**, **Magnus Emesenus**, *Iatrosophia*, (Hippocratis, Galeni, Magni et Erasistrati iatrosophium. Inc. Τὴν περὶ τῆς τῶν οὔρων).

Paris, Bibl. Nationale, Parisin. 2330; s. XV.

(f. 16ᵛ *und* 23ᵛ) *De urinis.*

Paris, Bibl. Nationale, Parisin. 2332; s. XIV, XIV (XV), XV (XIV), XV.
See **[2332]** below (p. 82).

De atra bile (Frgm.).
De crisibus libri III (Frgm.).
De diebus decretoriis libri III (Frgm.).
De praegnotione ad Epigenem (Frgm.).
In Hippocratis librum de acutorum victu commentarii IV (Frgm.).
Hippocratis aphorismi et Galeni in eos commentarii VII (Frgm. ex libr. I–VI).
Synopsis librorum suorum sedecim de pulsibus (Frgm. Exc. e l. περὶ σφυγμῶν).
(f. 6) *De temperamentis* (Frgm.).
(f. 6) *De differentiis morborum* (Frgm.).
(f. 6) *De morborum causis* (Frgm.).
(f. 6) *De symptomatum differentiis* (Frgm.).
(f. 6) *De locis affectis libri VI* (Frgm.).

(f. 130 [?]) *De pulsibus* (Frgm.).
(f. 199ᵛ) *De propriis placitis* (Frgm. Inc. Ἐδείχθη. Expl. νομίζουσιν).
(f. 401) *De differentiis febrium libri II* (de febribus liber I).

[Paris, Bibl. Nationale, Parisin. 2332; s. XIV, XV (XIV)].
Same as **2332** above (p. 81) (*Census*: 244, nr [1277]).

(f. 6) *Ars medica* (Frgm.).
(f. 6) *De elementis secundum Hippocratem* (Frgm.).

Paris, Bibl. Nationale, Parisin. 2333; s. XVI.

Ars medica.

Paris, Bibl. Nationale, Parisin. 2383; s. XVI.

Scholia in Galenum.
(f. 7) *De fasciis.*
(f. 27–34ᵛ) *De iis, quae medice scripta sunt in Platonis Timaeo, fragmentum* (Sine auctoris nomine).

Paris, Bibl. Nationale, Parisin. 2494; s. XV.

(f. 258–260ᵛ) *Prognostica* (Προγνωστικὸν περὶ ἀνθρώπου. Inc. Συνέστηκεν ὁ κόσμος ἐκ δ' στοιχείων. Expl. εἰς τὰ μέλη ὅλου τοῦ σώματος. *Vgl.* Costomiris, Rev. des ét. gr. II [1889] p. 308 sq.).

Paris, Bibl. Nationale, Parisin. 2510; a. 1384, s. XIV.

(f. 61) *De succedaneis liber.*
(f. 80) **Hippokrates**, **Galenos**, **Dioscurides**, *De animalibus marinis et terrestribus ad morbos curandos idoneis.*
(f. 108) **Galenos**, **Paulus Aegineta**, **Theophilus**, *Excerpta varia* (Pracepta medica et remedia varia).
(f. 133ᵛ) *Remedia.*

Paris, Bibl. Nationale, Parisin. 2664; s. XVI.
Possibly same as **2164** above (p. 68) (*Census*: 249, nr [1308]).

(f. 218) *De antidotis libri II.*

Paris, Bibl. Nationale, Parisin. 2760; s. XVI.

(f. 21) *De humoribus.*

Paris, Bibl. Nationale, Parisin. 2830; a. 1515.

(f. 175) *De pulsibus ad tirones.*

Paris, Bibl. Nationale, Parisin. 3035; s. XIV.

(f. 197) *An animal sit quod est in utero.*
(f. 209) *Synopsis librorum suorum sedecim de pulsibus* (Liber de pulsibus).
(f. 209–219) *De pulsibus* (Frgm.).
(f. 219ᵛ) *De urinis.*

Paris, Bibl. Nationale, Suppl.
Now Paris, Bibliothèque nationale de France, supplément grec

Paris, Bibl. Nationale, Suppl. 2; s. XVI.

In Hippocratis de humoribus librum commentarii III.

Paris, Bibl. Nationale, Suppl. 35; s. XV–XVI.

(f. 1) *Definitiones medicae.*
(f. 23ᵛ) *Introductio sive medicus.*
(f. 61) *De affectuum renibus insidentium dignotione et curatione liber.*
(f. 77) *De tremore, palpitatione, convulsione et rigore.*
(f. 93) *De purgantium medicamentorum facultatibus.*
(f. 98ᵛ) *De parvae pilae exercitatione.*
(f. 102) *Quod qualitates incorporeae sint.*
(f. 109) *Puero epileptico consilium.*
(f. 110ᵛ) *De morborum temporibus.*
(f. 121) *De totius morbi temporibus.*
(f. 129) *De substantia facultatum naturalium fragmentum.*
(f. 130ᵛ) *De cuiuslibet animi peccatorum dignotione atque medela.*
(f. 132ᵛ) *De respirationis usu.*
(f. 144) *De praenotione.*
(f. 166) *De sectis ad eos qui introducuntur.*
(f. 177ᵛ) *De tumoribus praeter naturam.*
(f. 185ᵛ) *De theriaca ad Pisonem liber.*
(f. 215ᵛ) *De theriaca ad Pamphilianum.*
(f. 219) *De antidotis libri II.*

Paris, Bibl. Nationale, Suppl. 292; s. XVII.

(f. 269) *Excerpta varia.*

Paris, Bibl. Nationale, Suppl. 446; s. X.
See also [**Wien, Hofbibliothek, Vindob. med. 19 (?)**] below (p. 115).

(f. 1) *Ad Glauconem de medendi methodo libri II.*
(f. 31ᵛ) *De febribus* (Ἀποσημείωσις πυρεκτικιούντων. Inc. Κατεκλίθη ὁ νοσῶν ἐν ἀρχῇ τῆς α' ἡμέρας. Expl. ἡνίκα πυρετοὶ ὦσιν ἐπὶ τῷ κάμνοντι).
(f. 31ᵛ) *De differentiis febrium libri II* (de febri).
(f. 33ᵛ) *Synopsis librorum suorum sedecim de pulsibus.*
(f. 33ᵛ) *De pulsibus ad Antonium* (Inscr. Ἑρμηνεία π. σφυγμῶν καὶ θεωρία. Inc. Ὁπόταν ἰατρὸς ἐπ' ἀρρώστῳ κληθῇ = K. XIX 633, 10. Expl. *wie im* [Oxford, Bodl.] Clarkian. [16 (18378)] [above p. 57]. Subscr. ζήτει πρ. Ἀντώνιον φιλομαθῆ).
(f. 70) *Definitiones medicae* (Inc. mutil. –σαντο τὰ κατὰ τὴν ἰατρικὴν = K. p. 348, 1).
(f. 91) *De urinis* (Π. τῶν κατὰ φύσιν οὔρων. Inc. Ἐπὶ τῶν πυρεκτικῶν μάλιστα νοσημάτων. Expl. θάνατον σημαίνουσιν · εἰ δὲ καὶ περὶ ...).
(f. 92) *De urinis compendium.*
(f. 95) *De pulsibus ad tirones.*

Paris, Bibl. Nationale, Suppl. 447; s. XIV.
Vindob. med. gr. 34 ist jetzt Parisin. Suppl. 447.
See **Wien, Hofbibliothek, Vindob. med. 34** below (p. 117).

(f. 1) *Hippocratis aphorismi et Galeni in eos commentarii VII.*
(f. 229) *In Hippocratis vel Polybi opus de salubri victus ratione privatorum commentarius.*

Paris, Bibl. Nationale, Suppl. 496; s. XVII.

Ars medica.

Paris, Bibl. Nationale, Suppl. 629; s. XIX.

(f. 59) *Synopsis librorum suorum sedecim de pulsibus* (Tract. de pulsibus).
(f. 59–65) *De pulsibus* (Frgm.).

Paris, Bibl. Nationale, Suppl. 634; s. XIV.

(f. 2ᵛ) *De sectis ad eos qui introducuntur.*
(f. 19–21ᵛ. 25. 26. 22ʳ) *De elementis secundum Hippocratem* (»Scholia in elementa Hipp. aliosque libros continens«. Inscr. *und* Inc. *wie im* Neapol.

[Bibl. Borbon. 229 (III D 15)] [above p. 54]. *Vgl.* Costomiris Rev. des ét. gr. II [1889] p. 371s. Kalbfleisch, Gal. de victu attenuante p. VII[i]. VIII).

(f. 19–26[v]) *Scholia in Galenum* (*Vgl.* Kalbfleisch, de victu atten. p. VIII).

(f. 22) *De temperamentis* (Frgm. »Scholia in temperamenta continens«).

(f. 23[v]. 26[v]) *De propriis placitis* (Frgm.).

(f. 28) *De ossibus ad tirones.*

(f. 39) *Ad Glauconem de medendi methodo libri II.*

(f. 64) *Remedia* (Περὶ καταπλασμάτων. Inc. Τῶν καταπλασμάτων τὰ μέν ἐστιν ἑψητά. Expl. ἄλφιτα τῷ λινοσπέρμῳ. Ed. Costomiris, Rev. des ét. gr. II [1889] p. 371).

(f. 65) *De tumoribus praeter naturam.*

(f. 75) *Ars medica.*

(f. 103) *De urinis* (De urinis ex Hippocrate et Galeno »Ist mit K. XIX 609 ff. nicht identisch.« Helmreich).

(f. 112) *De urinis compendium.*

(f. 117) *De probis pravisque alimentorum sucis.*

(f. 133–140) *De victu attenuante.*

(f. 142) *De alimentorum facultatibus libri III.*

(f. 257) *Methodi medendi libri XIV* (L. I–VI. XIII–XIV).

Paris, Bibl. Nationale, Suppl. 635; s. XIII.

(f. 3) *De marcore* (*Nur der Schluß von p. 700, 4 an*).

(f. 3[v]) *Institutio logica.*

(f. 12–23[v]) *Ad Gaurum quomodo animetur fetus.*

Paris, Bibl. Nationale, Suppl. 636; s. XVI.

(f. 3) *De remediis parabilibus libri III.*

Paris, Bibl. Nationale, Suppl. 681; s. XIII–XVI.

(f. 6) *De generatione.*

Paris, Bibl. Nationale, Suppl. 682; s. X–XIX, XI.

(f. 130) *De succedaneis liber.*

Paris, Bibl. Nationale, Suppl. 683; s. XV–XVIII, XVIII.

(f. 1[v]) *Excerpta varia.*

Paris, Bibl. Nationale, Suppl. 684; s. XV–XVIII.

(f. 5^{v}) *De remediis parabilibus libri III.*
(f. 211–266^{v}) *Iatrosophia* (Ἰ. ἐκλελεγμ. ἐκ τοῦ Γαλ. καὶ Ἱππ. καὶ ἄλλ. τινῶν. Inc. Ἐγὼ Γαληνὸς πεπειραμένος. Expl. μετὰ ὄξους ὀλίγον καὶ ὠφελεῖται. *Vgl.* Costomiris, Rev. des ét. gr. II [1889] p. 378).

Paris, Bibl. Nationale, Suppl. 727; s. XIX.

(f. 21–49) *Ad Gaurum quomodo animetur fetus.*
(f. 71) *De ossibus ad tirones.*

Paris, Bibl. Nationale, Suppl. 764; s. XIV.

(f. 1) *Excerpta varia.*
(f. 121) *Ad Glauconem de medendi methodo libri II.*
(f. 151) *De alimentorum facultatibus libri III.*

Paris, Bibl. Nationale, Suppl. 765; s. XVII.

De ossibus ad tirones.

Paris, Bibl. Nationale, Suppl. 793; s. XVII.

Indices in Galenum (Lud. Kusteri in Gal.).

Paris, Bibl. Nationale, Suppl. 1193; s. XVI.

(f. 17) *De antidotis libri II* (Frgm.).
(f. 17) *De succedaneis liber* (Frgm.).

Paris, Bibl. Nationale, Suppl. 1194; s. XV.

(f. 1) *Excerpta varia.*

Paris, Bibl. Nationale, Suppl. 1202; s. XIII, XIII–XVI, XIV–XVI.

(f. 16) **Archigenes, Dioscurides, Galenos, Magnus Emesenus, Oribasius, Paulus Aegineta, Porphyrius, Socrates,** *Excerpta varia* (Excerpta varia ex Diosc., Oribas., Porphyrio, Paulo, Magno, Archigene etc.).

Paris, Bibl. Nationale, Suppl. 1297; s. XI.

De succedaneis liber.

Petersburg, Kaiserl. öffentl. Bibl.
Санкт-Петербург (Sankt-Peterburg [Saint Petersburg]), Российская Национальная Библиотека, Санкт-Петербург (Rossiiskaia Natsional'naia Biblioteka, Sankt-Peterburg [National Library of Russia, Saint Petersburg])

Petersburg, Kaiserl. öffentl. Bibl., 116; a. 1318.

(f. 214ᵛ) *Iatrosophia* (Ἰ. ἐκ τῶν Γαλ. εἰς πᾶν εἶδος ὠφέλιμον).

Pistoia

Pistoja, Biblioteca Fabroniana, 141 (308); s. XVI.
Now Pistoia, Biblioteca Capitolare Fabroniana, Ms 308 (*Census*: 266, nr [1409]).

(f. 1) *Hippocratis aphorismi et Galeni in eos commentarii VII.*
(f. 146) *In Hippocratis prognosticum commentarii III.*

Ravenna

Ravenna, Biblioteca Classens., 70; s. XV.
See also **131, 2, H** below.

Opera varia.

Ravenna, Biblioteca Classens., 131, 2, H; s. XV.
Same as **70** above.
= Ms. 70 (*Census*: 267, nr [1413]).

Ars medica.
Introductio sive medicus.

Rom, Bibl. Angelica
Roma, Biblioteca Angelica

Rom, Bibl. Angelica, 17 (C.5. 4); s. XIV.
Now Ang. gr. 17 (*Census*: 270, nr [1419]).

(f. 9) *De non intentis* (Inc. Ἀνέντατον ποιῆσαι καὶ συνουσίας).
(f. 51ᵛ) *Remedia* (κατ' ἀλφαβήτου. σπε'. ἀλφοὺς μέλανας ἀποκαθαίρει).

Rom, Bibl. Barberin.
Now at Città del Vaticano, Biblioteca Apostolica Vaticana, *Barberiniani*

Rom, Bibl. Barberin., I 5; s. XV.
Now *Vaticanus Barberinianus graecus* 5 (*Census*: 272, nr [1422]).

(f. 1) **Hippokrates**, *Aphorismi* (c. comm. Gal.; Expl. θανάσιμον τὸ τοιοῦτον).

Rom, Bibl. Barberin., I 80 (= 273); s. –, XV.
Now *Vaticanus Barberinianus graecus* 80 (*Census*: 272, nr [1428]).

(f. 1) *De ossibus ad tirones.*
(f. 42) *De septimestri partu.*

Rom, Bibl. Barberin., I 118; s. IV, XIV, XV.
Now *Vaticanus Barberinianus graecus* 118 (*Census*: 273, nr [1430]).

(f. 262) *De ossibus ad tirones.*

Rom, Bibl. Barberin., I 127; s. XVI.
Now *Vaticanus Barberinianus graecus* 127 (*Census*: 273, nr [1431]).

(f. 1^{v}) *De pulsibus* (Inc. *wie im* Lond. Medical Society H Hi 17 [above p. 38]. Expl. οὐ χαλεπῶς εὑρήσετε).
(f. 189^{v}) *Prognostica de decubitu ex mathematica scientia.*
(f. 207) *Lexicon botanicum* (Inc. Ἀβρότονον. Expl. ὑπάρχει δυνάμεως).
(f. 251) *De pulsibus* (Inc. *wie im* Lond. Medical Society H Hi 17. Expl. ἐν τοῖς καρποῖς παρείς).
(f. 255) *De gynaeceis i. e. de passionibus mulierum* (Inc. Μήτρα λέγεται καὶ ὑστέρα. Expl. in cap. περὶ τῶν δίμηνα καὶ τρίμηνα φθειρουσῶν· πρὸς τὰς μὴ συλλαμβανούσας).
(f. 261^{v}) *Introductio sive medicus* (Frgm. Inc. Ὅτι παρὰ τῷ Γαλ. πρῶτος Ἀπόλλων ἐφεῦρεν ἰατρικήν. Expl. τῶν εἰσφερομένων κοινοτήτων θεωρία).
(f. 262) *De urinis* (Inc. *wie im* Lond. [Brit. Mus.] Addit. 17, 900 [above p. 36]. Expl. κατάλυσιν τῆς σαρκός).
(f. 278^{v}) *De pulsibus* (Inc. Πῶς ἐνεστῶσαν κρίσιν. Expl. ὄγκοι γίγνοιντο. Sine auctoris nomine).

Rom, Bibl. Barberin., I 152; s. XVI.
Now *Vaticanus Barberinianus graecus* 152 (*Census*: 273, nr [1432]).

(f. 39) *De septimestri partu.*

Rom, Bibl. Barberin., III 63 (= 245); s. XVI.
Now *Vaticanus Barberinianus graecus* 344 (*Census*: 273, nr [1434]).

(f. 394–414^{v}) **Hippokrates**, **Galenos**, **Meletius monachus**, *Jatrosophium* (Ἰατροσόφιον ἐκλελεγμένον Γαλ. Ἱππ. καὶ Μελετίου περὶ γυναικός. Expl. εἰς τὰ νευροχαλαστικά).

Rom, Bibl. Corsiniana (= Acc. d. Lincei)
Now Roma, Biblioteca Corsiniana, Accademia dei Lincei

Rom, Bibl. Corsiniana (= Acc. d. Lincei), 1410 (36. E. 26); s. –.
Now *Corsin.* 36.E.26 (1410) (*Census*: 274, nr [1441]).

(f. 344) *Remedia* (Ἀλάτιον Γαλ.).
(f. 385) *De urinis* (Inc. *wie im* Scorial. Υ. III. 14 [above p. 19]. Expl. καὶ τῆς γενομένης προρρήσεως θεωρεῖν).

Rom, Bibl. St. Petri

Rom, Bibl. St. Petri, H 45; s. XIII.
Now Città del Vaticano, Biblioteca Apostolica Vaticana, Archivio di San Pietro H 45 (*Census*: 275, nr [1443]).

Opera varia (»Palimpsest very damaged contains Galen; part of his works«. Allen).

Rom, Bibl. Vallicellana
Roma, Biblioteca Vallicelliana

Rom, Bibl. Vallicellana, 21 (B 93); s. XIV.
Now B 93 (*Census*: 276, nr [1446]).

(f. 65^{v}) *Quod animi mores corporis temperamenta sequantur.*

Rom, Bibl. Vaticana, Ottobon.
Now Città del Vaticano, Biblioteca Apostolica Vaticana, *Ottoboniani*

Rom, Bibl. Vaticana, Ottobon. 311; s. XV–XVI, XVI.

(f. 28) *De differentiis febrium libri II.*
(f. 28 [*hinter*]) *De facultatibus naturalibus* (Frgm. Π. φύσεως δυνάμεων κεφάλαια).
(f. 28 [*hinter*]) *De temperamentis.*
(f. 112) *Definitiones medicae.*

Rom, Bibl. Vaticana, Palat.
Now Città del Vaticano, Biblioteca Apostolica Vaticana, *Palatini*

Rom, Bibl. Vaticana, Palat. 31; s. XIV.

(f. 1) *De simplicium medicamentorum temperamentis et facultatibus libri XI* (Lib. III init. mut. – VI. IX–XI. Lib. XI lacunos.).

Rom, Bibl. Vaticana, Palat. 54; s. XV–XVI.

(f. 1) *Ad Glauconem de medendi methodo libri II.*
(f. 24) *De locis affectis Libri VI.*
(f. 103ᵛ) *De compositione medicamentorum secundum locos libri X.*
(f. 341) *De differentiis febrium libri II.*

Rom, Bibl. Vaticana, Palat. 128; s. XV.

(f. 1) *Ars medica.*
(f. 26ᵛ) *Hippocratis aphorismi et Galeni in eos commentarii VII* (in aph. XIV primos).

Rom, Bibl. Vaticana, Palat. 143; s. XV.

(f. 164) *De victus ratione in morbis acutis ex Hippocratis sententia* (Inc. Μελίκρητον δὲ πινόμενον. »Spectare videntur ad Gal. libr. de victus ratione in morb. acut., ex Hipp. sententia.«).
(f. 167) *Praesagitio omnino vera expertaque.*
(f. 172) *De morborum temporibus.*
(f. 173) *De urinis.*
(f. 175ᵛ) *Qua ratione adiuvandi ii sint, qui remedio hausto non purgantur.*
(f. 176) *Remedia* (Helleborus quibusdam sit dandus).

(f. 177) *Remedia* (Inc. Ἀγάλλοχον τὸ μὲν σῶμα).
(f. 178^{v}) *Excerpta varia* (Inc. Περὶ δὲ τῶν τεκμηρίων).

Rom, Bibl. Vaticana, Palat. 157; s. XIV.

(f. 1) *De differentiis febrium libri II* (Frgm. de febribus).
(f. 1) *De febribus.*
(f. 2 [= 2^{v}]) *In Hippocratis prognosticum commentarii III.*
(f. 110) *De crisibus libri III.*
(f. 219) *De diebus decretoriis libri III.*

Rom, Bibl. Vaticana, Palat. 173; s. XV.
= ? *Vaticanus Reginensis* 173 below (p. 94) (*Census*: 279, nr [1474]).

(f. 1) *In Hippocratis prognosticum commentarii III.*

Rom, Bibl. Vaticana, Palat. 199; s. XIII.

(f. 2^{v}) *Excerpta varia.*
(f. 3) *De simplicium medicamentorum temperamentis et facultatibus libri XI* (Frgm. De lacte ex libro IV).
(f. 4^{v}) *De sectis ad eos qui introducuntur* (Expl. νῦν δὲ εἰσαγομένοις ἱκανὰ ταῦτα. [M. W.]).
(f. 7) *Ars medica* (Frgm.).
(f. 11) *De differentiis febrium libri II.*
(f. 15^{v}) *De succedaneis liber* (Inc. Τὸ συνώνυμον ἀρχὴ τοῦ α' ἀντὶ ἀκανθίου σπέρματος λυχνίς. Expl. ἀντὶ ὠκιμοειδοῦς ἡδύοσμον ἄγριον. [M. W.]).
(f. 84) *De alimentorum facultatibus libri III* (Libri II. In fine catal. herbar. purgantium. Expl. κἄπειτα προελθόντων ἡμῶν = K. VI 599, 6).
(f. 183^{v}) *De optima corporis nostri constitutione* (Inscr. ρκδ' λόγος · ὧν [l. ὃν] ἐποίησαν Ἱπποκράτης καὶ ὁ μετ' αὐτοῦ [sic] Γαληνὸς καὶ περὶ φυσικῆς ἀκροάσεως. Inc. *wie im* [Flor.] Laurent. 74, 10 [above p. 23] [M. W.]).
(f. 186) *Excerpta varia* (Περὶ πυρετῶν καὶ ἄλλων τινῶν · ἐκ τῶν Γαληνοῦ. 10 Kapitel. Inc. Μετὰ τὴν τῶν ὑγιεινῶν. Expl. τῆς ἀρίστης ἡλικίας τοῦ λείποντος ἡ δύναμις [M. W.]).
(f. 192 sq.) *Definitiones medicae* (Frgm. Inc. Γαληνοῦ [in mg.] περὶ μὲν τῶν νοσημάτων τῶν συμβαινόντων τοῖς ἀνθρώποις τὰ μέν ἐστι συνεχῆ, τὰ δὲ διαλείποντα = Gal. XIX 387 K. [M. W.]).
(f. 471) *Quos, quibus catharticis medicamentis et quando purgare opporteat* (Frgm.).

Rom, Bibl. Vaticana, Palat. 251; s. XV.

(f. 1) *De usu partium corporis humani libri XVII.*

Rom, Bibl. Vaticana, Palat. 278; s. XIV–XV.

(f. 31ᵛ) *Hippocratis aphorismi et Galeni in eos commentarii VII* (in sectiones VI).

Rom, Bibl. Vaticana, Palat. 279; s. XIV–XV.

(f. 21ᵛ) *De venae sectione* (Inc. *wie im* Lond. [Brit. Mus.] Add. [17, 900] [above p. 36]).
(f. 31ᵛ) **Hippokrates**, *Aphorismi* (sectt. duae primae c. scholiis; sectiones VI c. comm. Galeni).
(f. 213ᵛ) *De venae sectione* (Inc. Διηγήσατό ποτε).
(f. 266) *De succedaneis liber* (Inc. *wie im* Lond. [Brit. Mus.] Addit. [10, 058] [above p. 36]).
(f. 277) *Remedia* (de medicamentis stomacho idoneis. Inc. Ἅπερ ἀεὶ λέγω).
(f. 307) *De crisibus libri III* (Frgm.).
(f. 311) *De hominis natura testamentum. De victu singulis mensibus servando* (Inc. *wie im* Athous Διονυσίου [3701. 167] [above p. 6]).

Rom, Bibl. Vaticana, Palat. 295; s. XV–XVI.

(f. 177) *De crisibus libri III* (Frgm. Exc. e ll. II et III).
(f. 187) *De corporis partibus* (Frgm Galeni; Inc. Ὁ δὲ γαργαρεὼν ὃν καὶ σταφύλην καλέουσι).

Rom, Bibl. Vaticana, Palat. 297; s. XV–XVI.

De febribus (De febrium substantia et differentiis. Inc. Σκοπὸν οὖν ἔχομεν. *Vgl.* Palladius *bei* Ideler, Phys. et med. I p. 107).
Excerpta varia.
(f. 19ᵛ) *Definitiones medicae.*
(f. 50) *De sectis ad eos qui introducuntur* (Frgm. »de Empiricis et Methodicis«).

Rom, Bibl. Vaticana, Palat. 385; s. XV–XVI.

(f. 1) *Hippocratis aphorismi et Galeni in eos commentarii VII* (init. et fine mutil.).

Rom, Bibl. Vaticana, Palat. 400; s. XV.

(f. 7) **Hippokrates**, **Galenos**, *De febribus* (Ex Hipp. et Gal. de febribus. Inc. Ἱπποκράτης ὁ διδάσκαλος ἡμῶν).
(f. 7) *De differentiis febrium libri II* (Frgm. Inc. Ἱπποκράτης ὁ διδάσκαλος ἡμῶν).
(f. 48) *De pulsibus ad tirones.*
(f. 68) *De venae sectione.*
(f. 399) *Remedia* (de prophylacticis adversus arthricos affectus).

Rom, Bibl. Vaticana, Palat. 428; s. XV–XVI, XV–XVII.

(f. 1) *Index* (Index in Gal., Alex. Aphr. et Hipp. aliquot opuscola).
(f. 1) *De urinis* (Inc. Πλεῖον κουφίζει εἰς τόν).

Rom, Bibl. Vaticana, Passioneian. Now Città del Vaticano, Biblioteca Apostolica Vaticana, *Rossianus*

Rom, Bibl. Vaticana, Passioneian. 2; s. –.
Now *Vaticanus Rossianus* 982 (*Census*: 274–275, nr [1442]).
See also Wien, **Bibl. Colleg S. J. Rossianus, XI.167** below (p. 112).

De usu partium corporis humani libri XVII (Libri XVI).

Rom, Bibl. Vaticana, Reg. Suec. Now Città del Vaticano, Biblioteca Apostolica Vaticana, *Reginenses*

Rom, Bibl. Vaticana, Reg. Suec. 154; s. XV.
Vatic. 154 = Reg. Suec. 154; vgl. J. v. Müller, Galeni Scripta minora II p. XXXIV.
See **Vatic. 154** below (p. 96).

(f. 1) *Ars medica.*
(f. 41) *Quod animi mores corporis temperamenta sequantur.*

Rom, Bibl. Vaticana, Reg. Suec. 172; s. XIV.

(f. 1v) *De compositione medicamentorum per genera libri VII.*
(f. 105) *De compositione medicamentorum secundum locos libri X.*
(f. 229) *De ponderibus et mensuris* (Sine auctoris nomine).

Rom, Bibl. Vaticana, Reg. Suec. 173; s. XV.
See also (possibly) **Palat. 173** above (p. 91) and **[Vatic. ap. Montfauc. p. 28]** below (p. 96).

(f. 73) *De antidotis libri II.*
(f. 73ᵛ) *In Hippocratis librum de acutorum victu commentarii IV.*
(f. 185) *Galeni in Hippocratis de natura hominis lib. commentarii II.*
(f. 222) *In Hippocratis vel Polybi opus de salubri victus ratione privatorum commentarius.*
(f. 233) *De sanitate tuenda libri VI.*
(f. 355ᵛ) *De ptisana.*

Rom, Bibl. Vaticana, Reg. Suec. 174; s. XIV.

(f. 1) *Methodi medendi libri XIV.*

Rom, Bibl. Vaticana, Reg. Suec. 175; s. XIV.
See also (possibly) **[Vatic. ap. Montfaucon p. 34]** below (p. 96).

(f. 1 [= 2ʳ]) *In Hippocratis prognosticum commentarii III.*
(f. 89) *In Hippocratis praedictionum librum primum commentarii III.*
(f. 179ᵛ) *De difficultate respirationis libri III.*
(f. 240ᵛ) *De causis respirationis.*
(f. 242) *De motu musculorum libri II.*

Rom, Bibl. Vaticana, Reg. Suec. 181; a. 1364.

(f. 225) *De pulsibus ad tirones* (Frgm. Inc. Ἐν τοῖς σφυγμοῖς μόνον τοῦ καρποῦ).
(f. 285) *De urinis.*

Rom, Bibl. Vaticana, Urbin.
Now Città del Vaticano, Biblioteca Apostolica Vaticana, *Urbinates*

Rom, Bibl. Vaticana, Urbin. 64; s. X–XI, XIII.

(f. 48ᵛ) **Galenos** (*Ist der Commentar des* Palladius *unter den Namen des* Galen), *Scholia in Hippocratis de popularibus morbis librum sextum, sectiones VIII* (Σχόλιον τῆς ἕκτης ἐπιδημίας ἀπὸ φωνῆς Γαλ. VII partes. Inc. Ἄρτι ταῖς μεθόδοις τὰ ὀξέα τῶν νοσημάτων).

Rom, Bibl. Vaticana, Urbin. 65; s. XIV.

(f. 1) *Hippocratis aphorismi et Galeni in eos commentarii VII.*

Rom, Bibl. Vaticana, Urbin. 67; s. XIII, XIV, XIV–XV, XV.

(f. 1) *Introductio sive medicus.*
(f. 33) *In Hippocratis de humoribus librum commentarii III.*
(f. 53) *De compositione medicamentorum secundum locos libri X.*
(f. 188) *De simplicium medicamentorum temperamentis et facultatibus libri XI* (Libri VI–XI).
(f. 268) *De remediis parabilibus libri III* (Liber I).
(f. 276) *Quod optimus medicus sit etiam philosophus* (Expl. λαβόντι μὴ οὐχὶ καὶ τὰς ἄλλας).
(f. 282) *De simplicium medicamentorum temperamentis et facultatibus libri XI* (Libri I–V).

Rom, Bibl. Vaticana, Urbin. 68; s. XIV.

(f. 3) *Linguarum sive dictionum exoletarum Hippocratis explicatio.*

Rom, Bibl. Vaticana, Urbin. 69; s. X–XI.

(f. 1) *De usu partium corporis humani libri XVII* (Expl. f. 195^{v} προβάλλοντες = K. 364, 19).

Rom, Bibl. Vaticana, Urbin. 70; s. XV.

(f. 1) *De alimentorum facultatibus libri III* (Inc. a l. I c. 7; in fine addit. remedium π. καθαρτηρίων).
(f. 64) *De venae sectione adversus Erasistrateos Romae degentes.*
(f. 80) *De venae sectione adversus Erasistratum.*
(f. 90) *De curandi ratione per venae sectionem.*
(f. 104) *De theriaca ad Pamphilianum.*
(f. 107) *De melancholia ex Galeno, Rufo, Posidonio et Marcello Sicamii Aetii libellus.*
(f. 107) *De atra bile* (Frgm. *Unter demselben Titel wie im* [Venet.] Marc. 279) (below p. 104).

Rom, Bibl. Vaticana, Vatic.
Now Città del Vaticano, Biblioteca Apostolica Vaticana, *Vaticani graeci*

[Rom, Bibl. Vaticana, Vatic. apud Montfauc. p. 28].
= ? *Vaticanus Reginensis graecus* 173 above (p. 94) (*Census*: 286, nr [1514]).

De natura hominis.

[Rom, Bibl. Vaticana, Vatic. ap. Montfaucon p. 34].
= ? *Vaticanus Reginensis graecus* 175 above (p. 94) (*Census*: 286–287, nr [1515]).

De animalibus (de motu animalium).

Rom, Bibl. Vaticana, Vatic. 154; s. XVI.
(= Reg. Suec. 154).
Same as **Reg. Suec. 154** above (p. 93).

Quod animi mores corporis temperamenta sequantur.

Rom, Bibl. Vaticana, Vatic. 269; s. XV.
= ? *Vaticanus graecus* 296 below (p. 98) (*Census*: 289–290, nr [1520]).

(f. 476) *De ponderibus et mensuris.*

Rom, Bibl. Vaticana, Vatic. 277; s. XIV.

(f. 12) *Linguarum sive dictionum exoletarum Hippocratis explicatio.*

Rom, Bibl. Vaticana, Vatic. 279; s. –, XII.
Verbleib unbekannt.
See *Census*: 290–291, nr [1524].
See also **Vatic. 1028** below (p. 98).

(f. 31) *Hippocratis aphorismi et Galeni in eos commentarii VII.*
(f. 213) *De venae sectione.*
(f. 237) *De succedaneis liber* (Π. ἀντ. καὶ ἐκ τῶν λέξεων βοταν.).
(f. 237) *Lexicon botanicum* (Frgm.).

Rom, Bibl. Vaticana, Vatic. 280; s. XV.

(f. 1) *Hippocratis aphorismi et Galeni in eos commentarii VII.*
(f. 158 [?]) *De urinis.*
(f. 158v) *De urinis* (Περὶ οὔρων πονηρῶν. Τί δηλοῦσιν αἱ πιτυρώδεις στάσεις. Inc. Ὅταν δὲ δαπανήσει).

(f. 159) *De urinis* (Π. τῶν κατὰ φύσιν οὔρων. Inc. *wie im* Scorial. Υ. III. 14) (above p. 19).

Rom, Bibl. Vaticana, Vatic. 281; s. XIV.

(f. 30v) *De pulsuum differentiis libri IV.*
(f. 42) *De dignoscendis pulsibus libri IV.*
(f. 73v) *De causis pulsuum libri IV.*
(f. 106) *De praesagitione ex pulsibus libri IV.*

Rom, Bibl. Vaticana, Vatic. 282; s. XV.
s. XVI.

De facultatibus naturalibus.
(f. 1) *De elementis secundum Hippocratem.*
(f. 15) *De temperamentis.*
(f. 46v) *De inaequali intemperie.*
(f. 50) *De facultatibus naturalibus.*
(f. 87) *De crisibus libri III* (»Mit Lücken im 2. und 3. Buche.« M. W.).
(f. 121) *De diebus decretoriis libri III.*

Rom, Bibl. Vaticana, Vatic. 283; s. XIV.

(f. 1v) *Quomodo morbum simulantes sint deprehendi.*
(f. 1) *De dignotione ex insomniis.*
(f. 2) *De hirudinibus, revulsione, cucurbitula, incisione et scarificatione.*
(f. 12) *De dignotione ex insomniis.*
(f. 12v) *De praenotione.*
(f. 20) *De tumoribus praeter naturam.*
(f. 22) *Hippocratis aphorismi et Galeni in eos commentarii VII.*

Rom, Bibl. Vaticana, Vatic. 284; s. XI–XII (?), XII.
s. XI.

De simplicium medicamentorum temperamentis et facultatibus libri XI (Vorn unvollständig; enthält B. VI–XI mit Dioscurides περὶ ὕλης ἰατρικῆς verarbeitet [M. W.]).

Rom, Bibl. Vaticana, Vatic. 285; s. XV.

(f. 49) *Introductio sive medicus.*
(f. 81) *De morborum temporibus* (Περὶ τῶν ἐν παροξυσμοῖς καιρῶν).
(f. 92) *De totius morbi temporibus.*

(f. 110) *De tremore, palpitatione, convulsione et rigore.*
(f. 112) *Ars medica.*
(f. 127) *De uteri dissectione.*
(f. 133) *Puero epileptico consilium.*
(f. 139) *De atra bile.*
(f. 153) *De differentiis febrium libri II.*
(f. 202ᵛ) *De dignotione ex insomniis.*
(f. 209) *De usu partium corporis humani libri XVII* (Lib. I–III cap. 9).

Rom, Bibl. Vaticana, Vatic. 296; s. XV.
See also (possibly) **Vatic. 269** above (p. 96).

(f. 476) *De succedaneis liber.*

Rom, Bibl. Vaticana, Vatic. 300; s. XII–XIII.

(f. 287ᵛ–288ᵛ) *De diebus decretoriis libri III* (Inc. Τὰ νοσήματα ἅτινα. Expl. καὶ τοῦ γνῶναι τὰ σημεῖα).

Rom, Bibl. Vaticana, Vatic. 695; s. XIV–XV.

(f. 226) *De hominis natura* (Περὶ τῆς συστάσεως τοῦ ἀνθρώπου).

Rom, Bibl. Vaticana, Vatic. 1028; s. –.
= V*aticanus graecus* 279, ff. I–III, above (p. 96) (*Census*: 296–297, nr [1557]).

(f. I) *Methodi medendi libri XIV* (« Lib. X c. 10 vel ex hoc capite »).

Rom, Bibl. Vaticana, Vatic. 1063; s. XIII.

(f. 1) *In Hippocratis prognosticum commentarii III* (Der Anfang des Commentars ist verloren gegangen. Anfang = K. XVIII B 46).
(f. 107ᵛ) *De dignotione ex insomniis.*
(f. 109) *De praenotione.*
(f. 114ᵛ) *Quomodo morbum simulantes sint deprehendi.*

Rom, Bibl. Vaticana, Vatic. 1064; s. –.

(f. 25ᵛ) *De pulsuum differentiis libri IV.*
(f. 114) *De dignoscendis pulsibus libri IV.*
(f. 141) *De causis pulsuum libri IV* (Libri III ?).
(f. 201) *De praesagitione ex pulsibus libri IV.*

Rom, Bibl. Vaticana, Vatic. 1066; s. XVI.
s. XV.

(f. 78 [= 78r]) *Prognostica de decubitu ex mathematica scientia.*
(f. 168) *De simplicium medicamentorum temperamentis et facultatibus libri XI* (διαγνώσεις ex libro I).
(f. 169) *De simplicium medicamentorum temperamentis et facultatibus libri XI* (Liber II).

Rom, Bibl. Vaticana, Vatic. 1444; s. XVI.
See *Census*: 300, nr [1576].

(f. 22v) *Prognostica de decubitu ex mathematica scientia* (K. XIX p. 529–571).
(f. 223) *De chirurgorum operationibus et de decubitu infirmorum.*

Rom, Bibl. Vaticana, Vatic. 1595; s. IX.

(f. 200) *De succedaneis liber* (Frgm. *Vgl.* H. Schoene, Mitteilungen zur Geschichte der Medizin 1902, 141).

Rom, Bibl. Vaticana, Vatic. 1614; s. XVI.

(f. 122) *Definitiones medicae.*

Rom, Bibl. Vaticana, Vatic. 1692 B; s. XV.
= *Vaticanus graecus* 1702 (*Census*: 301, nr [1581]).

(f. 7) *Prognostica de decubitu ex mathematica scientia.*

Rom, Bibl. Vaticana, Vatic. 1700; s. XIV.

(f. 27v) *De hominis natura testamentum. De victu singulis mensibus servando* (Δίαιτα ἀκριβὴς π. καταστάσεως ὑγιεινῆς τοῦ ἀνθρώπου καὶ τῆς κατασκευῆς αὐτοῦ).

Rom, Bibl. Vaticana, Vatic. 1845; s. XIII.

Ars medica (Frgm. Inc. γνώρισμα τῆς ἐν πνεύμονι = K. I 350, 5. Expl. τῶν ἰδίων συγγραμμάτων, *vgl.* K. I 412).
(f. 44v) *Introductio sive medicus.*
(f. 106) *De morborum temporibus* (Inscr. *wie im* Vatic. [gr.] 285 [above p. 97]).
(f. 122v) *De totius morbi temporibus.*
(f. 133) *De uteri dissectione.*
(f. 142v) *Puero epileptico consilium.*

(f. 152) *De atra bile.*
(f. 171v) *De tremore, palpitatione, convulsione et rigore.*
(f. 197v) *De praegnotione ad Epigenem.*

Rom, Bibl. Vaticana, Vatic. 1858; s. –.

(f. 234) *In Hippocratis prognosticum commentarii III* (Inc. Ὅτι μὲν ἀντί. Expl. εὐθέως ὁμολογουμένου ὡς τα …).

Rom, Bibl. Vaticana, Vatic. 1898; s. –.

(f. 65. 66. 67) *De ponderibus et mensuris.*
(f. 67) *De succedaneis liber.*

Rom, Bibl. Vaticana, Vatic. 2182; s. XV.

(f. 48) *Ad Glauconem de medendi methodo libri II* (Lib. I in fine mutil.; des. τῆς ἡμέρας ἡ μὲν = K. XI 66).

Rom, Bibl. Vaticana, Vatic. 2254; s. X–XI.

(f. 1) *Ad Glauconem de medendi methodo libri II.*

Rom, Bibl. Vaticana, Vatic. 2256; s. XIV.
See *Census*: 305, nr [1601].

(f. 33) *De succedaneis liber.*
(f. 78v) *De urinis* (Inc. *und* Expl. *wie im* [Oxon.] Laudian. [58] [above p. 58]).
(f. 79v) *Remedia* (πρὸς δυσεντερικούς).

Rom, Bibl. Vaticana, Vatic. lat. 5763; s. V–VI.

(f. 30v) *De alimentorum facultatibus libri III* (*Palimpsest; vgl. Sitz. Ber. d. Berl. Ak. 1902 p. 442 f.* Inc. ἔλλοβα = K. VI 557, 11. Expl. οὐ μὴν ἐπί γε = K. VI 559, 4).

Rosanbo

Rosanbo, Bibl. de M. le marquis de Ros., 286; s. XVI.

(f. 90) *De compositione medicamentorum secundum locos libri X* (τῶν εἰς ι' τὸ δέκατον. Περὶ νεφριτικῶν. Inc. Ὅτι μὲν νεφριτικάς. Expl. ἀναλάμβανε …).

Turin, Bibl. Nazionale (Universitaria)
Now Torino, Biblioteca Nazionale Universitaria

Turin, Bibl. Nazionale (Universitaria), Taurin. – (« zitiert bei Montfaucon, 1837, 'Galenos de IV elementis'; nicht verifiziert).
Possibly B. V. 39 (*Census*: 318, nr [1622]).

De elementis secundum Hippocratem.

Turin, Bibl. Nazionale (Universitaria), Taurinens. 6 b IV 6; s. XVI.
See also **6 b IV 6 (B I 6)** below.
Now B. I. 6 (*Census*: 318, nr [1623]).

De morbis Excerpta (»fort. Galeni«).

Turin, Bibl. Nazionale (Universitaria), Taurin. 6 b IV 6 (B I 6); s. XVI.
Same as **6 b IV 6** above.
= B. I. 6 (*Census*: 318, nr [1624]).

(f. 185) *De venae sectione* (Inc. *wie im* Monacens. [39] [above p. 51].
(f. 191) *De alimentorum facultatibus libri III*.
(f. 230^{v}) *De alimentorum facultatibus libri III* (*Wie im* Monac. 39, f. 86).

Upsala, Upsal. bibl. acad.
Now Uppsala Universitet

Upsala, Upsal. bibl. acad., 8 (e don. Jo. Gabr. Sparfwenf. 49); s. –, XV.
Now Gr 8 (*Census*: 320, nr [1635]).

Lexicon botanicum (*Ob von Galen, ist fraglich*).

Upsala, Upsal. bibl. acad., nr. 25; s. XVI.
Now Gr 25 (*Census*: 321, nr [1636]).

(f. 39^{v}) *De propriorum animi cuiuslibet affectuum dignotione et curatione* (Frgm. Inc. *und* Expl. *wie im* Bernens. 691 [above p. 12]).

Venedig, Monast. S. Michaelis prope Murianum/ Bibl. monaster. S. Michaelis Venet. prope Murianum

Venedig, Monast. S. Michaelis prope Murianum, 93; s. XVI.
Verbleib unbekannt.
Same as **London, British Museum, Addit. 6898** above (p. 36) (*Census*: 326, nr [1651]).
= London, British Library, Additional 6898.

Methodi medendi libri XIV (Ἀπὸ θεραπευτικῆς ἐκ τοῦ περὶ τραυμάτων. Inc. πῶς τὸ πύον γίνεται λευκόν – τὰ δὲ συμπτώματα ἐν ταῖς ἐνεργείαις · σχολ. τὸ περὶ διαφορᾶς πυρετῶν).

Venedig, Bibl. monaster. S. Michaelis Venet. prope Murianum, 132; s. –.
Verbleib unbekannt.
Same as **Berlin, Königl. Bibl., Hamilton. 270 (401)** above (p. 10) (*Census*: 326–327, nr [1652]).
= Berlin, Staatsbibliothek zu Berlin – Preussischer Kulturbesitz SBB-PKB, Ms. Ham. 270.

De placitis Hippocratis et Platonis libri IX (Libri VII; desunt primus et initium secundi libri).

Venedig, Bibl. Nazionale Marciana, Marcian. Now Venezia, Biblioteca Nazionale Marciana, *Marciani graeci*

[Venedig, Bibl. Nazionale Marciana, Marcian.].
Possibly *graecus* 269 (coll. 533) below (*Census*: 327, nr [1654]).

In librum Hippocratis de aetatum aegritudinibus.

Venedig, Bibl. Nazionale Marciana, graecus, 269; s. XI.
Now *graecus* 269 (coll. 533) (*Census*: 329, nr [1662]).
See also (possibly) **[Marcian.]** above.

Linguarum sive dictionum exoletarum Hippocratis explicatio.

Venedig, Bibl. Nazionale Marciana, graecus, 275; s. XV.
Now *graecus* 275 (coll. 893) (*Census*: 330, nr [1669]).

De facultatibus naturalibus.
(f. 1) *Ars medica.*

(f. 31) *De elementis secundum Hippocratem.*
(f. 56ᵛ) *De temperamentis.*
(f. 176ᵛ) *De differentiis morborum.*
(f. 190) *De morborum causis.*
(f. 202ᵛ) *De symptomatum differentiis.*
(f. 215) *De symptomatum causis libri III.*

Venedig, Bibl. Nazionale Marciana, graecus, 276; s. XII.
Now *graecus* 276 (coll. 917) (*Census*: 330, nr [1670]).
See also **[276]** below.

De sanitate tuenda libri VI.
(f. 68) *De marcore.*
(f. 74) *Methodo medendi libri XIV.*
(f. 261) *De atra bile.*
(f. 268) *De causis respirationis* (Expl. εἶθ' ἑκάτερον αὐτῶν = K. IV 468, 6).
(f. 268) *De oculis* (Frgm. Γαλ. περὶ τῶν ἐν τοῖς ὀφθαλμοῖς παθῶν διάγνωσις. Inc. Ὀφθαλμοὶ νοσοῦσιν. »Nur 6 Zeilen, die aber mitsamt dem Titel von derselben Hand wieder durchgestrichen worden sind« Schoene).
(f. 269) *De parvae pilae exercitatione.*

[Venedig, Bibl. Nazionale Marciana, graecus, 276].
Same as **276** above.
= *graecus* 276 (coll. 917) (*Census*: 330, nr [1671]).

De melancholia ex Galeno, Rufo, Posidonio et Marcello Sicamii Aetii libellus (Π. φλεβοτομίας. » Hic codex deest«; *Verwechselung mit dem* Palat. 279 ?).

Venedig, Bibl. Nazionale Marciana, graecus, 277; a. 1416, s. XV.
Now *graecus* 277 (coll. 630) (*Census*: 330, nr [1672]).

In Hippocratis vel Polybi opus de salubri victus ratione privatorum commentarius (sine titulo).
Hippocratis aphorismi et Galeni in eos commentarii VII.

Venedig, Bibl. Nazionale Marciana, graecus, 278; s. XI.
Now *graecus* 278 (coll. 873) (*Census*: 330, nr [1673]).

(f. 1) *Hippocratis aphorismi et Galeni in eos commentarii VII.*
(f. 146) *In Hippocratis vel Polybi opus de salubri victus ratione privatorum commentarius.*

Venedig, Bibl. Nazionale Marciana, graecus, 279; s. XV.
Now *graecus* 279 (coll. 705) (*Census*: 330, nr [1674]).
See also **[279 (?)]** below.

(f. 1) *De anatomicis administrationibus libri IX.*
(f. 71–84v) *De motu musculorum libri II.*
(f. 84v–130v) *In Hippocratis de articulis librum commentarii IV.*
(f. 130v–163v) *In Hippocratis librum de fracturis commentarii III.*
(f. 163v–202) *In Hippocratis librum de officina medici commentarii III.*
(f. 205–243) *De alimentorum facultatibus libri III.*
(f. 253–258v) *De venae sectione adversus Erasistrateos Romae degentes.*
(f. 259–267v) *De curandi ratione per venae sectionem.*
(f. 267v–269v) *De theriaca ad Pamphilianum.*
(f. 269v–271) *De melancholia ex Galeno, Rufo, Posidonio et Marcello Sicamii Aetii libellus.*
(f. 269v–271) *De atra bile* (Frgm. Περὶ μελαγχολίας ἐκ τῶν Γαλ. καὶ Ῥούφου καὶ Ποσειδωνίου, in marg. τοῦ Ἀετίου. Inc. Ὥσπερ ἐν τοῖς φαινομένοις μέλεσιν. Expl. στυπτηρίαν ἐπιπάσομεν τῷ ὄξει).

[Venedig, Bibl. Nazionale Marciana, graecus, 279 (?)].
Same as **279** above.
Now *graecus* 279 (coll. 705) (*Census*: 330–331, nr [1675]).

De venarum arteriarumque dissectione.

Venedig, Bibl. Nazionale Marciana, graecus, 280; s. XV.
Now *graecus* 280 (coll. 706) (*Census*: 331, nr [1676]).

De compositione medicamentorum secundum locos libri X.
(f. 1–22v) *Ad Glauconem de medendi methodo libri II.*
(f. 24–102) *De locis affectis Libri VI.*

Venedig, Bibl. Nazionale Marciana, graecus, 281; s. XV.
Now *graecus* 281 (coll. 581) (*Census*: 331, nr [1677]).

De propriorum animi cuiuslibet affectuum dignotione et curatione.
(f. 2–46v) *In Hippocratis librum de acutorum victu commentarii IV.*
(f. 47–71v) *In Hippocratis praedictionum librum primum commentarii III.*
(f. 72–75v) *De pulsibus ad tirones.*
(f. 75v–76v) *De substantia facultatum naturalium fragmentum* (Inc. *wie* im [Mediolan.] Ambros. [Q 3 Sup.] [above p. 42]).
(f. 76v–77) *De cuiuslibet animi peccatorum dignotione atque medela* (Expl. νῦν εἶναι μόνην).

(f. 77v–81v) *De respirationis usu.*
(f. 81v) *De praegnotione ad Epigenem.*
(f. 81v) *De praenotione* (Π. τοῦ προγινώσκειν).
(f. 89) *De totius morbi temporibus.*
(f. 91) *De tumoribus praeter naturam.*
(f. 93v) *De theriaca ad Pisonem liber.*
(f. 104v) *De theriaca ad Pamphilianum.*
(f. 106) *De antidotis libri II.*

Venedig, Bibl. Nazionale Marciana, graecus, 282; s. XV.
Now *graecus* 282 (coll. 648) (*Census*: 331, nr [1678]).
See also [**282**] below.

De affectuum renibus insidentium dignotione et curatione liber.
De atra bile.
De bono habitu.
De inaequali intemperie.
De marcore.
De optima corporis nostri constitutione.
De sectis ad eos qui introducuntur.
De tremore, palpitatione, convulsione et rigore.
Galeni in Hippocratis de natura hominis lib. commentarii II.
In Hippocratis vel Polybi opus de salubri victus ratione privatorum commentarius.
(f. 1) *Puero epileptico consilium.*
(f. 3) *De morborum temporibus.*
(f. 3) *De sanitate tuenda libri VI.*
(f. 6v–33) *De crisibus libri III.*
(f. 33–53v) *De diebus decretoriis libri III.*
(f. 53v–85v) *In Hippocratis prognosticum commentarii III.*
(f. 85v) *De differentiis febrium libri II.*
(f. 199v–200v) *De parvae pilae exercitatione.*

[Venedig, Bibl. Nazionale Marciana, graecus, 282].
Same as **282** above.
Now *graecus* 282 (coll. 648) (*Census*: 331, nr [1679]).

De melancholia ex Galeno, Rufo, Posidonio et Marcello Sicamii Aetii libellus (*Verwechselung wie bei* [Venet. Marcian.] nr. 276 [above p. 103]).

Venedig, Bibl. Nazionale Marciana, graecus, 283; s. XV.
Now *graecus* 283 (coll. 631) (*Census*: 331, nr [1680]).

(f. 1) *In Hippocratis epidemiarum libros commentarii* (in libr. VI).

Venedig, Bibl. Nazionale Marciana, graecus, 284; s. XV.
Now *graecus* 284 (coll. 707) (*Census*: 331, nr [1681]).
See also **[284]** below.

De atra bile.
De parvae pilae exercitatione.
De placitis Hippocratis et Platonis libri IX (»Libri VII sine primo«).
Methodo medendi libri XIV (»stammt aus Marc. 276.« [above p. 103] M. W.).

[Venedig, Bibl. Nazionale Marciana, graecus, 284].
Same as **284** above.
Now *graecus* 284 (coll. 707) (*Census*: 332, nr [1682]).

De melancholia ex Galeno, Rufo, Posidonio et Marcello Sicamii Aetii libellus (*Verwechselung wie bei* [Marcian.] nr. 276).

Venedig, Bibl. Nazionale Marciana, graecus, 285; s. XV.
Now *graecus* 285 (coll. 708) (*Census*: 332, nr [1683]).

In Hippocratis vel Polybi opus de salubri victus ratione privatorum commentarius.
Hippocratis aphorismi et Galeni in eos commentarii VII.
In Hippocratis epidemiarum libros commentarii (in libr. III).
(f. 128–211^{v}) *De compositione medicamentorum per genera libri VII* (Expl. μάλιστα χειμῶνος ἔν γε ταῖς ὁ = K. XIII 1052, 18).
(f. 244) *De probis pravisque alimentorum sucis.*

Venedig, Bibl. Nazionale Marciana, graecus, 286; s. XV.
Now *graecus* 286 (coll. 626) (*Census*: 332, nr [1684]).

De simplicium medicamentorum temperamentis et facultatibus libri XI.

Venedig, Bibl. Nazionale Marciana, graecus, 287; s. XV.
Now *graecus* 287 (coll. 709) (*Census*: 332, nr [1685]).

(f. 1–155^{v}) *De usu partium corporis humani libri XVII.*
(f. 157–196) *De pulsuum differentiis libri IV.*
(f. 196^{v}–224^{v}) *De dignoscendis pulsibus libri IV.*
(f. 225–253) *De causis pulsuum libri IV.*
(f. 254–287) *De praesagitione ex pulsibus libri IV.*

Venedig, Bibl. Nazionale Marciana, graecus, 288; s. X.
s. XI.
Now *graecus* 288 (coll. 913) (*Census*: 332, nr [1686]).

De compositione medicamentorum secundum locos libri X.
De ponderibus et mensuris.

Venedig, Bibl. Nazionale Marciana, graecus, 295; a. 1470, s. XIV.
s. XIV falso pro a. 1470 (M. W.).
Now *graecus* 295 (coll. 729) (*Census*: 333, nr [1693]).

(f. 179–186ᵛ) *De succedaneis liber* (Expl. ἰμίσυος κυπρίου.

Venedig, Bibl. Nazionale Marciana, graecus, 336; s. XV, XV–XVI.
Now *graecus* 336 (coll. 646) (*Census*: 333, nr [1700]).

(f. 251ᵛ) *Prognostica de decubitu ex mathematica scientia* (Expl. ἀναιρεθήσονται γάρ).

Venedig, Bibl. Nazionale Marciana, graecus, 509; s. XV.
Now *graecus* 509 (coll. 845) (*Census*: 333, nr [1702]).

Excerpta varia.

Venedig, Bibl. Nazionale Marciana, appendix graeca
Now Venezia, Biblioteca Nazionale Marciana, *appendix graeca*

Venedig, Bibl. Nazionale Marciana, appendix graeca, II, 171; s. XV.
Now *app. gr.* II.171 (coll. 445) (*Census*: 334, nr [1708]).

De hirudinibus, revulsione, cucurbitula, incisione et scarificatione (Frgm.).
De venae sectione (Π. φλεβοτομίας. Inc. Ἀπὸ μὲν τῶν ὁμοιομερῶν. Expl. τμητικοῖς ἰώμεθα *und* Τίς καιρὸς φλεβοτομίας).

Venedig, Bibl. Nazionale Marciana, appendix graeca, V, 4; s. XV.
Now *app. gr.* V.4 (coll. 544) (*Census*: 335, nr [1713]).

Ad Glauconem de medendi methodo libri II.
Adversus ea quae Juliano in Hippocratis aphorismos enuntiata sunt libellus (»Unvollständig«. Helmreich.).
Adversus Lycum.
An animal sit quod est in utero.

An in arteriis natura sanguis contineatur.
De anatomia (Π. ἀνατ. τῶν ἐντὸς καὶ ἐκτός).
De anatomicis administrationibus libri IX (Περὶ ἀνατομῆς τῶν ἐντὸς καὶ τῶν ἐκτός).
De crisibus libri III.
De diebus decretoriis libri III.
De differentiis morborum.
De foetuum formatione.
De instrumento odoratus.
De morborum causis.
De purgantium medicamentorum facultatibus.
De symptomatum causis libri III.
De symptomatum differentiis.
De temperamentis.
In Hippocratis librum de acutorum victu commentarii IV.
Methodi medendi libri XIV.
Quod optimus medicus sit etiam philosophus.
Quod qualitates incorporeae sint.
(f. 242) *De parvae pilae exercitatione.*
(f. 256) *Thrasybulus sive utrum medicinae sit an gymnastices hygieine.*
(nr 11) *De septimestri partu.*

Venedig, Bibl. Nazionale Marciana, appendix graeca, V, 5; s. XV.
Now *app. gr.* V.5 (coll. 1053) (*Census*: 335, nr [1714]).

(f. 2) *Hippocratis aphorismi et Galeni in eos commentarii VII.*
(f. 89) *In Hippocratis librum de acutorum victu commentarii IV.*
(f. 145) *Prognostica* (Prologus de prognosticis in morbis acutis. Inc. Σκοπός ἐστιν ἐνταῦθα τῷ).
(f. 145ᵛ) *In Hippocratis prognosticum commentarii III.*
(f. 182ᵛ) *In Hippocratis praedictionum librum primum commentarii III* (Commentarius duplex).
(f. 222) *De difficultate respirationis libri III.*
(f. 249) *In Hippocratis epidemiarum libros commentarii* (in libr. II.).
(f. 311) *In Hippocratis epidemiarum libros commentarii* (in libr. III. libri II.).
(f. 313) *De symptomatum causis libri III.*
(f. 322) *De atra bile.*
(f. 328) *De purgantium medicamentorum facultatibus.*
(f. 330ᵛ) *De praenotione.*
(f. 333ᵛ) *Quomodo morbum simulantes sint deprehendi.*
(f. 334ᵛ) *Quos, quibus catharticis medicamentis et quando purgare opporteat.*

(f. 336^{v}) *De locis affectis libri VI.*
(f. 332^{v}) *De dignotione ex insomniis.*
(f. 394^{v}) *De plenitudine.*
(f. 403) *De morborum temporibus* (inscr. *wie im* Vatic. [gr.] 285). (above p. 97).
(f. 407) *De totius morbi temporibus.*
(f. 410^{v}) *De uteri dissectione.*
(f. 413^{v}) *Puero epileptico consilium.*
(f. 416) *De atra bile.*
(f. 421) *De tremore, palpitatione, convulsione et rigore.*
(f. 428) *De urinis.*
(f. 431) *De urinis* (Π. διαφορᾶς οὔρων. Inc. Ἐπὶ τῶν πυρετικῶν μάλιστα. Expl. προβαίνειν τὴν νόσον).
(f. 431^{v}) *Ars medica* (Capita quattuor prima; expl. κατὰ τὴν ἀρετὴν τῶν ἐνεργειῶν).
(f. 433) *De causis respirationis.*
(f. 433^{v}) *De motu musculorum libri II* (Expl. ταῖς ἡμέραις ὁ ἄνθρωπος = K. IV 443).

Venedig, Bibl. Nazionale Marciana, appendix graeca, V, 6; s. XIII.
Now *app. gr.* V.6 (coll. 1207) (*Census*: 335, nr [1715]).

(p. 199) *De simplicium medicamentorum temperamentis et facultatibus libri XI.*

Venedig, Bibl. Nazionale Marciana, appendix graeca, V, 7; s. XIV.
Now *app. gr.* V.7 (coll. 1054) (*Census*: 335, nr [1716]).

(f. 1) *De compositione medicamentorum secundum locos libri X* (Libri III init. mutil.–X).

Venedig, Bibl. Nazionale Marciana, appendix graeca, V, 8; s. XIV.
Now *app. gr.* V.8 (coll. 1334) (*Census*: 335, nr [1717]).

(f. 10) *De crisibus libri III.*
(f. 62) *De diebus decretoriis libri III.*

Venedig, Bibl. Nazionale Marciana, appendix graeca, V, 9; s. XV.
Now *app. gr.* V.9 (coll. 1017) (*Census*: 335, nr [1718]).

(f. 1) *Hippocratis aphorismi et Galeni in eos commentarii VII* (Expl. ἵδρως πολύς = K. XVIII A 176).
(f. 131) *De morborum temporibus.*
(f. 139^{v}) *De totius morbi temporibus.*
(f. 145^{v}) *De uteri dissectione.*

(f. 150v) *Puero epileptico consilium.*
(f. 155) *De atra bile.*
(f. 164) *De tremore, palpitatione, convulsione et rigore.*
(f. 179) *Ars medica.*
(f. 206v) *Introductio sive medicus* (Expl. τὰ ἕλκη σπουδάζομεν.
(f. 366) *De simplicium medicamentorum temperamentis et facultatibus libri XI* (L. I–V).
(f. 469) *Excerpta varia* (Γαλ. περὶ τόπων πεπονθότων. Inc. Διάγνωσις τῶν πεπονθότων τόπων γίνεται ἢ ἀπὸ συμπτωμάτων. [M. W.]).
(f. 471) *Excerpta varia* (Γαλ. περὶ φυσικῶν δυνάμεων. Inc. Ἐν τούτῳ τῷ λόγῳ περὶ τῶν φυσικῶν μέλλει διδάξαι πλατύτερον. [M. W.]).
(f. 492) *De sectis ad eos qui introducuntur* (Expl. μετὰ ἀκριβείας).
(f. 500–507v) *Definitiones medicae* (Ohne Namen. Περὶ ὅρων διαφόρων εἰδῶν · τί ἐστι διάφραγμα; διάφραγμά ἐστι νευρῶδες διεῖργον καὶ χωρίζον τά τε ἐν τῷ θώρακι = Gal. XIX 360 K. Expl. f. 507v ἄφθα ἐστὶν ἕλκωσις ἐπιπόλαιος ἐν στόματι γινομένη · ἐπιπλάττει [sic] δὲ αὕτη ἡ ἕλκωσις μάλιστα παιδίοις = Gal. XIX 441 K. [M. W.]).
(f. 508) *Sermo adversus empiricos medicos* (Inc. ἢ σπανίως ἢ ἀμφιδόξως = p. 1263, 2 Sch. Expl. *wie im* [Mediol.] Trivult. [685] [above p. 44]).
(f. 508) *In Hippocratis librum de acutorum victu commentarii IV.*
(f. 514) *De usu partium corporis humani libri XVII* (Libri III–XVII; expl. ἥλιον ἢ σελήνην ἤ τινα τῶν ...).

Venedig, Bibl. Nazionale Marciana, appendix graeca, V, 10; s. XVI.
Now *app. gr.* V.10 (coll. 1444) (*Census*: 335, nr [1719]).

(f. 2) *Introductio sive medicus.*
(f. 29) *Hippocratis aphorismi et Galeni in eos commentarii VII.*
(f. 39) *Excerpta varia.*

Venedig, Bibl. Nazionale Marciana, appendix graeca, V, 11; s. XVI.
Now *app. gr.* V.11 (coll. 1064) (*Census*: 335, nr [1720]).

(f. 1) *De alimentorum facultatibus libri III* (Inc. mut. = K. VI 483, 13).

Venedig, Bibl. Nazionale Marciana, appendix graeca, V, 12; s. X–XIII.XV.
Now *app. gr.* V.12 (coll. 1317) (*Census*: 335, nr [1721]).

(f. 38) *De usu partium corporis humani libri XVII* (unum fol. Inc. ἐνέργεια μὲν οὖν μορίου. Expl. κατασκευῆς διαλέγεται »Hat mit Galen nichts zu tun«. Helmreich.).
(f. 144v) *De morborum causis* (Inscr. Περὶ αἰτίας παθῶν).

Venedig, Bibl. Nazionale Marciana, appendix graeca, V, 13; s. XIV–XVI.
Now *app. gr.* V.13 (coll. 1221) (*Census*: 336, nr [1723]).

(f. 119) *Excerpta varia*.

Venedig, Bibl. Nazionale Marciana, appendix graeca, V, 15; s. XVI.
Now *app. gr.* V.15 (coll. 1299) (*Census*: 335, nr [1727]).

In Hippocratis epidemiarum libros commentarii (in libr. I. liber I; Expl. τῶν ἔνδον τοῦ περιτοναίου μορίων; *Das* Expl. *ist vielmehr das von* Comm. III in Epid. Γ'; *vgl. oben* Monac. 231).

Venedig, Bibl. Nazionale Marciana, appendix graeca, V, 18; s. –.
Now *app. gr.* V.18 (coll. 985) (*Census*: 335, nr [1729]).

Excerpta varia (Ed. Aldina Gal. cuius in margine notae scriptae sunt).

Venedig, Bibl. Nazionale Marciana, appendix graeca, V, 19; s. –, XV.
Now *app. gr.* V.19 (coll. 986) (*Census*: 335, nr [1730]).

Excerpta varia (Ed. Aldina Gal. cuius in margine notae scriptae sunt).

Venedig, Bibl. Nazionale Marciana, appendix graeca, V, 20; s. –.
Now *app. gr.* V.20 (coll. 987) (*Census*: 335, nr [1731]).

Excerpta varia (Ed. Aldina Gal. cuius in margine notae scriptae sunt).

Venedig, Bibl. Nazionale Marciana, appendix graeca, V, 21; s. –.
Now *app. gr.* V.21 (coll. 988) (*Census*: 336, nr [1732]).

Excerpta varia (Ed. Aldina Gal. cuius in margine notae scriptae sunt).

Venedig, Bibl. Nazionale Marciana, appendix graeca, V, 22; s –.
Now *app. gr.* V.22 (coll. 989) (*Census*: 336, nr [1733]).

Excerpta varia (Ed. Aldina Gal. cuius in margine notae scriptae sunt).

Venedig, Bibl. Nazionale Marciana, appendix graeca, XI, 5; s. XIV.
Now *app. gr.* XI.5 (coll. 1254) (*Census*: 336, nr [1734]).

(f. 92) *De diebus decretoriis libri III*.

Warschau

Warschau, Bibl. Zamoyski, 142; s. XIII (?).
Warszawa, Biblioteka Narodowa, BN BOZ 142 (*Census*: 346, nr [1740]).

Ars medica.

Wien, Bibl. Colleg. S. J. Rossianus

Wien, Bibl. Colleg. S. J. Rossianus, XI.167; s. XV.
Now *Vaticanus Rossianus* 982 (*Census*: 348, nr [1742]).
See also **Rom, Bibl. Vaticana, Passioneian. 2** above (p. 93).

(f. 147v) *Remedia* (Σκευασία τῆς ἱερᾶς Γαληνοῦ εἰς φλεγματικοὺς καὶ μελαγχολικούς. Inc. κολοκυνθίδος οὐγγίας δ'. Expl. εἰς ἀποβροχὴν τῶν ὀπῶν).

Wien, Hofbibliothek, Vindob./Vindobon. Now Wien, Österreichische Nationalbibliothek, *Vindobonenses*

[Wien, Hofbibliothek, ap. Lambec. I 181].
= Wien, Österreichische Nationalbibliothek, Cod. Hebr. 29 (*Census*: 349–350, nr [1744]).

De crisibus libri III.
De facultatibus naturalibus.
De marcore.

[Wien, Hofbibliothek, ap. Lamb. II, c. 6].
Same as **Wien, Hofbibliothek, Vindob. med. 8** below (p. 114) (*Census*: 350, nr [1745]).
= Wien, Österreichische Nationalbibliothek, *medicus graecus* 8.

De compositione medicamentorum secundum locos libri X (L. VI–VIII).

[Wien, Hofbibliothek, Vindob. Lambec. VI p. 93].
Same as **Wien, Hofbibliothek, Vindob. med. 25** below (p. 115) (*Census*: 351, nr [1747]).
= Wien, Österreichische Nationalbibliothek, *medicus graecus* 25.

Excerpta varia.

[Wien, Hofbibliothek, Lambec. VI p. 100].
Same as **Wien, Hofbibliothek, Vindob. med. 15** below (p. 114) (*Census*: 351, nr [1748]).
= Wien, Österreichische Nationalbibliothek, *medicus graecus* 15.

Excerpta varia.

[Wien, Hofbibliothek, Lambec. VI p. 151].
Same as **Wien, Hofbibliothek, Vindob. med. 16** below (p. 115) (*Census*: 352, nr [1750]).
= Wien, Österreichische Nationalbibliothek, *medicus graecus* 16.

Excerpta varia (Anon. tabulae divisionum in plusculis libris Gal.).

[Wien, Hofbibliothek, Lambec. VI p. 153].
Same as **Wien, Hofbibliothek, Vindob. med. 13** below (p. 114) (*Census*: 352, nr [1751]).
= Wien, Österreichische Nationalbibliothek, *medicus graecus* 13.

Excerpta varia.

[Wien, Hofbibliothek, Vindob. ap. Nessel P. III].
Same as **Wien, Hofbibliothek, Vindob. med. 15** below (p. 114) (*Census*: 354, nr [1755]).
= Wien, Österreichische Nationalbibliothek, *medicus graecus* 15.

In Hippocratis librum de acutorum victu commentarii IV.

[Wien, Hofbibliothek, Vinddob. ap. Nessel III 27 (?) nr 5].
Same as **Wien, Hofbibliothek, Vindob. med. 16** below (p. 115) (*Census*: 354–355, nr [1756]).
= Wien, Österreichische Nationalbibliothek, *medicus graecus* 16.

De differentiis febrium libri II.

[Wien, Hofbibliothek, Vindob. ap. Nessel III 38 (?)].
Same as **Wien, Hofbibliothek, Vindob. med. 28** below (p. 116) (*Census*: 355, nr [1757]).
= Wien, Österreichische Nationalbibliothek, *medicus graecus* 28.

De differentiis febrium libri II.

Wien, Hofbibliothek, Vindob., 131; s. –.
Same as **Wien, Hofbibliothek, Vindob. med. 15** below (*Census*: 355, nr [1759]).
= Wien, Österreichische Nationalbibliothek, *medicus graecus* 15.
See also **[131]** below.

De morborum causis (Frgm.).

[Wien, Hofbibliothek, Vindob., 131].
Possibly same as **Wien, Hofbibliothek, Vindob. med. 15** below (*Census*: 356, nr [1760]).
= ? Wien, Österreichische Nationalbibliothek, *medicus graecus* 15.
See also **131** above.

De morbis Excerpta (Frgm. protheoriae de causis variorum morborum).

Wien, Hofbibliothek, Vindob. med. 1; s. V–VI, VI in., VI.

(f. 1) *De simplicium medicamentorum temperamentis et facultatibus libri XI* (*Vgl.* M. Wellmann, Hermes 38, 292–304).
(f. 1) *Lexicon botanicum* (Frgm.).

Wien, Hofbibliothek, Vindob. med. 8; s. XV.
See also **[ap. Lamb. II, c. 6]** above (p. 112).

(f. 318v) *Ars medica* (Expl. συστῆναι = K. I 312, 17).

Wien, Hofbibliothek, Vindob. med. 13; s. –, XV.
See also **[Lambec. VI p. 153]** above (p. 113).

Excerpta varia.
(f. 6v–23v) *Ad Glauconem de medendi methodo libri II* (Expl. εἰς μακρὸν κελεύειν καὶ τῶν σπλάγχνων προνοεῖσθαι κατανοοῦντά τε ...).

Wien, Hofbibliothek, Vindob. med. 15; s. –.
s. XV.
See **[Lambec.VI p. 100]** (p. 113), **[ap. Nessel P. III]** (p. 113), **Vindob., 131**, and possibly **[Vindob., 131]** above.

Excerpta varia.
(f. 138) *De propriis placitis* (Frgm. Inc. *und.* Expl. *wie im* Parisin. 2332). (above p. 81).

Wien, Hofbibliothek, Vindob. med. 16; s. XV–XVI.
s. XV.
See also **[Lambec. VI p. 151]** (p. 113) and **[ap. Nessel III 27 (?) nr 5]** (p. 113) above.

(f. 287) *Definitiones medicae.*
(f. 329) *Opera varia* (ἀρχὴ σὺν θεῷ τῶν διαιρέσεων πασῶν τῶν γαληνείων πραγματειῶν ἀρχόμενος ἀπὸ τοῦ περὶ αἱρέσεων, τελευτῶν δὲ εἰς τὴν θεραπευτικήν. Expl. ἢ διὰ τὰ συναμφότερα).

Wien, Hofbibliothek, Vindob. med. 18; s. –, XV, XVI.

(f. 1–256) *De locis affectis VI.*
(f. 2) *Ad Glauconem de medendi methodo libri II* (Frgm. Inc. οὐ δεῖται τὸ πλῆθος. Expl. εἰ δ' ἐξ ἀγενοῦς σίτου λαμβάνεις τὸ ἄλευρον).

[Wien, Hofbibliothek, Vindob. med. 19 (?)].
Now Paris, Bibliothèque nationale de France, *Supplementum graecum* 446 above (p. 84) (*Census*: 359, nr [1783]).

De urinis.

Wien, Hofbibliothek, Vindob. med. 20; s. XV.

(f. 484) *De succedaneis liber.*
(f. 486v–488) *Remedia* (Ἱερὰ Γαληνοῦ. Inc. Ἡ σύνθεσις ἔχει οὕτως. Expl. πίνειν μαλάχης σπέρματος ∠β' [sic !]).

Wien, Hofbibliothek, Vindob. med. 22; s. –, XV.

(f. 1–195) *De locis affectis libri VI.*

Wien, Hofbibliothek, Vindob. med. 25; s. XV, XV–XVI.
See **also [Lambec. VI p. 93]** above (p. 112).

(f. 11) *De simplicium medicamentorum temperamentis et facultatibus libri XI* (Frgm. ex libris VI–VIII).

Wien, Hofbibliothek, Vindob. med. 26; s. XV.

(f. 303) *De succedaneis liber.*

Wien, Hofbibliothek, Vindob. med. 28; s. –, XV.
See also **[Vindob. ap. Nessel III 38 (?)]** above (p. 113) and **med. [28 (?)]** below.

De praesagitione ex pulsibus libri IV (Θεοφίλου ἐκ τοῦ προγνωστικοῦ Γαλ. π. σφυγμῶν).
(f. 17ᵛ) *Methodi medendi libri XIV* (Frgm. Ἀπὸ θεραπευτικῆς ἐκ τοῦ περὶ τραυμάτων. Inc. πῶς τὸ πύον γίνεται λευκόν – τὰ δὲ συμπτώματα ἐν ταῖς ἐνεργείαις · σχολ. τὸ περὶ διαφορᾶς πυρετῶν).
(f. 184–185ᵛ) *De humoribus* (Inc. Ὁ κόσμος ἐκ δ' στοιχείων. Expl. καὶ ἡ διὰ τοῦ γάλακτος).
(f. 186ᵛ) *De venae sectione* (Inc. *wie im* Lond. [Brit. Mus.] Add. [17, 900] [above p. 36]. Expl. καὶ τῶν ἀλλοτρίων ἀποκριτικήν).

[Wien, Hofbibliothek, Vindob. med. 28 (?); s. XV].
Same as **28** above (*Census*: 360, nr [1793]).
= *medicus graecus* 28.

De succedaneis liber.

Wien, Hofbibliothek, Vindob. med. 29; s. XV.

(f. 12) *De venae sectione* (Inc. *wie im* Lond. [Brit. Mus.] Add. [17, 900] [above p. 36]. Expl. καθαρισμὸν τοῦ ἐγκεφάλου ἐξάγον).

Wien, Hofbibliothek, Vindob. med. 30; s. XV.

De dignotione ex insomniis (Frgm.).
(f. 475–477) *De laterum morbo ad Patrophilum* (Expl. δίδου μεσονύκτιος μετὰ σαχάρου).

Wien, Hofbibliothek, Vindob. med. 31; s. –, XV ex.
s. XV.

(f. 149–150) *Remedia.*

Wien, Hofbibliothek, Vindob. med. 32; s. XVI.

(f. 11) *De hominis natura testamentum. De victu singulis mensibus servando* (Διαθ. Γαλ. διδάσκουσα ἡμᾶς ἅπαντα κατ' ἀνθρωπίνου σώματος).
(f. 31) *De succedaneis liber* (Frgm. Inc. Ἀντὶ ἀμυγδάλου πικρὸν ἀψίνθιον. Expl. ἀντὶ ὠκίμου ἡδέος μονάγριον).

Wien, Hofbibliothek, Vindob. med. 34; s. –.
= Par. suppl. gr. 447.
Now Paris, Bibliothèque nationale de France, *Supplementum graecum* 447 above (p. 84) (*Census*: 360, nr [1798]).

In Hippocratis de natura hominis lib. commentarii II.
(f. 1) *Hippocratis aphorismi et Galeni in eos commentarii VII.*
(f. 229) *In Hippocratis vel Polybi opus de salubri victus ratione privatorum commentarius.*

Wien, Hofbibliothek, Vindob. med. 35; s. XV ex.

(f. 1–236v) *De simplicium medicamentorum temperamentis et facultatibus libri XI* (Libri VI–XI 2).

Wien, Hofbibliothek, Vindob. med. 37; s. –, XV.

Excerpta varia.

Wien, Hofbibliothek, Vindob. med. 41; s. XIV.
s. XIV–XV.

(f. 114–115) *Remedia.*

Wien, Hofbibliothek, Vindob. med. 44; s. XV.XVI, XV–XVI.

(f. 232) *In Hippocratis prognosticum commentarii III.*

Wien, Hofbibliothek, Vindob. med. 47; s. XV, XVI.

De urinis (Expl. *wie im* [Oxfon. Bodl.] Laudian. [58 (nunc 59; Bodl. 708)] [above p. 58]).
(f. 9) *Iatrosophia* (Ἰ. ... Γαλ. περὶ πάντων νοσημάτων).

Wien, Hofbibliothek, Vindob. med. 48; s. XIV–XV.

(f. 46–164) *De simplicium medicamentorum temperamentis et facultatibus libri XI* (Libri VI–VIII).
(f. 164v–171v) *De antidotis libri II* (Frgm. ex. l. I).

Wien, Hofbibliothek, Vindob. med. 52; s. –, XV.

(f. 23–35v) *De pulsibus ad tirones* (Expl. ὥστε καὶ μικρὸν εἶναι αὐτὸν καὶ ἀμυδρόν).

Wien, Hofbibliothek, Vindob. med. 53; s. XVI.

(f. 8^{v}–10^{v}) *De hominis natura testamentum. De victu singulis mensibus servando* (Wie im Athous Ξηροποτ. [2432. 99] [above p. 9]).
(f. 11–59) *Excerpta varia.*

Wien, Hofbibliothek, Vindob. phil. 178; s. XV.
Now *philos. et philol. gr.* 178 (*Census*: 362: nr [1823]).

(f. 25^{v}) *De urinis* (Π. οὔρων διὰ στοιχείων. Inc. α. ὑελίον βορβορῶδες. Expl. δηλοῖ τὴν φύσιν; Byzant. Werkchen).

Wien, Hofbibliothek, Vindob. phil. 303; s. XVI.
Now *philos. et philol. gr.* 303 (*Census*: 362: nr [1829]).

(f. 250–279^{v}) *Quod animi mores corporis temperamenta sequantur.*

Wolfenbüttel, Bibl. Guelf. August.
Now Wolfenbüttel, Herzog August Bibliothek Wolfenbüttel

Wolfenbüttel, Bibl. Guelf. August., Guelfberbyt. 837 (757 Helmst.); s. –.
Same as **Helmstad. 757.837** below (p. 120).
= 757 Helmst. (*Census*: 370, nr [1852]).

De propriorum animi cuiuslibet affectuum dignotione et curatrione.

Wolfenbüttel, Bibl. Guelf. August., Guelferb. 4148 (64 Weissenb.); s. –.
Same as **Weissenb. 64** below (p. 120).
= 64 Weiss. (*Census*: 371, nr [1854]).

De alimentorum facultatibus libri III (*Vgl.* K. Koch, Sitz.-Ber. d. Berl. Akad. 1907 p. 103–111).

Wolfenbüttel, Bibl. Guelf. August., Guelferbyt. 364 (Gud. 7 et 18); s. XVI.
= 7 and 8 Gud. lat. 2° (*Census*: 369, nr [1844]).
See also **Guelferbyt. Ebert 364 (7 und 8 Gud. lat.)** below (p. 119).

Opera varia (Aldina a. 1525 cum emendatt. Scaligeri marg. adscriptis).

Wolfenbüttel, Bibl. Guelf. August., Guelferbyt. Ebert 364 (7 und 8 Gud. lat.); s. XVI.
= 7 and 8 Gud. lat. 2° (*Census*: 369, nr [1841]).
See also **Guelferbyt. 364 (Gud. 7 et 18)** above (p. 118).

Opera varia.

Wolfenbüttel, Bibl. Guelf. August., Guelferb. Ebert. 368 (11 Gud. gr.); s. XVI.
Same as **Guelferb. 368 (Gud. 11)** below.
= 11 Gud. graec. fol. (*Census*: 370, nr [1845]).

De pulsibus ad tirones.
De pulsuum differentiis libri IV.

Wolfenbüttel, Bibl. Guelf. August., Guelferb. 368 (Gud. 11); s. XVI.
Same as **Guelferb. Ebert. 368 (11 Gud. gr.)** above.
= 11 Gud. graec. fol. (*Census*: 370, nr [1846]).

De pulsibus ad tirones.
De pulsuum differentiis libri IV (λόγος δεύτερος π. διαφορ. σφυγμ. Inc. Οὐ τὴν αὐτὴν χρή. Expl. mutil. κινδυνεύω δ' εἰπεῖν ὅτι τὸ τῶν πολλῶν).

Wolfenbüttel, Bibl. Guelf. August., Guelferbyt. 369 (Gud. 69); s. XVII.
= 69 Gud. graec. 4° (*Census*: 370, nr [1847]).
See also **Guelferbyt. Ebert. 369 (69 Gud. gr.)**, **Guelferbyt. 369. 370 (Gud. 69)**, and **Guelferb. Ebert. 370 (69 Gud. gr.)** below.

Methodi medendi libri XIV.

Wolfenbüttel, Bibl. Guelf. August., Guelferbyt. Ebert. 369 (69 Gud. gr.); s. XVII.
Same as **Guelferbyt. 369 (Gud. 69)** above.
= 69 Gud. graec. 4° (*Census*: 370, nr [1848]).

Methodi medendi libri XIV.

Wolfenbüttel, Bibl. Guelf. August., Guelferbyt. 369. 370 (Gud. 69); s. XVII.
Same as Guelferbyt. **369 (Gud. 69)** above.
= 69 Gud. graec. 4° (*Census*: 370, nr [1849]).

Ad Glauconem de medendi methodo libri II.

Wolfenbüttel, Bibl. Guelf. August., Guelferb. Ebert. 370 (69 Gud. gr.); s. XVII.
Same as Guelferbyt. **369 (Gud. 69)** above.
= 69 Gud. graec. 4° (*Census*: 370, nr [1850]).

Ad Glauconem de medendi methodo libri II.

Wolfenbüttel, Bibl. Guelf. August., Helmstad. 757.837; s. XVI.
= 757 Helmst. (*Census*: 370, nr [1851]).
See also **Guelfberbyt. 837 (757 Helmst.)** above (p. 118).

De propriorum animi cuiuslibet affectuum dignotione et curatione.

Wolfenbüttel, Bibl. Guelf. August., Weissenb. 64; s. V–VI.
= 64 Weiss. (*Census*: 371, nr [1853]).
See also **Guelferb. 4148 (64 Weissenb.)** above (p. 118).
Palimpsest.

(f. 43–57, 67–74, 82–89, 98–105, 114–137, 146–153, 162–169,186–193, 218–225, 268–270, 273–275, 305–310) *De alimentorum facultatibus libri III.*

Zeitz

Zeitz, Stiftsbibliothek, Cizens. 66; s. XVI.
Now Stiftsbibliothek und Stiftsarchiv Zeitz.

(f. 100–116) *Quod animi mores corporis temperamenta sequantur.*

www.ingramcontent.com/pod-product-compliance
Ingram Content Group UK Ltd.
Pitfield, Milton Keynes, MK11 3LW, UK
UKHW050953290926
15470UKWH00006B/1799

9 783110 600681